Don't Fear the Big Dogs

Journey to Loma Linda

Bill Vancil

TATE PUBLISHING, LLC

Don't Fear the Big Dogs/ Journey to Loma Linda
by Bill Vancil

This book is designed to provide accurate and authoritative information with regard to the subject matter covered. This information is given with the understanding that neither the author nor Tate Publishing, LLC is engaged in rendering legal, professional advice. Since the details of your situation are fact dependent, you should additionally seek the services of a competent professional.

ISBN: 1-9332903-7-4

Foreword

There is in everyone's life, a turning point. A moment or a season that becomes a sort of historical hinge: when all that had been, no longer was, and everything that was possible, became. For Bill Vancil, the "moment" came packaged in a thunderbolt; a bullet-to-the-bone diagnosis that would change his life forever.

When Vancil was told he had prostate cancer, he raced to find a cure for his illness, and a direction toward which to travel. In the process, in an unexpected time and place, he found the symmetry that was his life.

Don't Fear the Big Dogs is a story replete with discovery; a look at all our lives, seen through the moments and the miles of an incredible journey.

This book is a rich dessert of a story, woven like vines through Bill's sixty-third year, just as the sunlit back roads of southern California mapped his journey with thirteen year old daughter, Tori Lou.

Together they logged over seven thousand miles. They cried, they laughed, they sang songs, and discovered each other all over again.

Bill's pilgrimage was like a hike up the misty trails of a precipitous gorge ... shrouded in fog, tentatively climbing ... when suddenly the fog lifts, giving way to a verdant geometry below, under blue skies and a snow-capped mountain's magnificent, shimmering detail. It was that way for Bill Vancil and his daughter in the sun-and-honey days that stretched across the summer of 2004.

Arguably the story of someone seeking remedy from a serious illness or a life setback is not singularly unusual. There are in fact, countless epics of uplifting deliverance from near tragedy; each deserving of the telling.

What differentiates Bill's story bubbles to the top through his boundless awakening along the journey where child becomes parent, and parent–just for a little while–becomes child.

Bill left Madison, Wisconsin bound for Loma Linda University Medical Center looking for a cancer cure. He found so much more on the main roads and back roads of southern California and beyond.

Sometimes there's a golden story that captures a golden time; never to be again. In this uplifting account, Bill finds his cure and a hidden map to greater happiness. It's impossible to read these chapters without being inspired–without being a part of an incredible journey.

Ride with Bill and Tori Lou with the top down, racing before the canyon wind. You'll laugh, you'll cry, and you may – just for a fleeting moment – see yourself in the mirror, discovering. . .

Tim Moore

Managing Partner,
Audience Development Group
East Grand Rapids, Michigan
Author of *"The Motivator"*

Preface

The two of us were trying to shoehorn just one more briefcase into the trunk of my car. We hadn't worried about trunk size when we chose the convertible. All we thought about was how much we'd enjoy driving with the top down while in California.

"It's not going to fit Dad," said Tori Lou, in her junior-adjutant voice.

I was hearing her sound more and more grown up lately, more sure of herself and unabashed in courteously expressing her opinions. I wasn't entirely ready for her ascension into adolescence.

"Now I think if we can cram it this way, then back," I offered.

"It still won't go," she responded, without a moment's hesitation.

That's the way kids are today; so much more certain of just about everything, while we parents are less sure of just about anything.

We decided to put the remaining briefcase on the floor of the back seat. "It won't blow out of the car, Dad. It's too heavy. Your external hard drive is in there," my omniscient daughter reminded me.

That's how it began; a sunny Sunday morning in Wisconsin, May 9th, 2004. Me in my sixty-third year, capably advised by my thirteen-year-old daughter, preparing to drive solo on the first leg of the journey of our lives–well–*my* life to be sure.

Ten weeks earlier, as winter melted into spring, I heard the disquieting news from my doctor: "Bill, your PSA score is fairly high. I'm referring you to a urologist."

"You have prostate cancer," the urologist later confirmed. "We need to decide what to do."

In the buzz and blur, within which I suddenly became enveloped, a voice from the far corner of my being reminded me that my life story was about to change inexorably, with the ending incomplete. All bets off . . . no dues left to pay.

What mattered yesterday was not on today's top one-hundred list. I was suddenly standing at the intersection of, *Why Me & To Hell with This.*

I said goodbye to Tori Lou, at this point knowing I would not see her for about two months. After a long hug, which seemed short, I aimed the convertible toward California and drove off, sobbing all the way to Cedar Rapids.

Three months later there we were - Bill and Tori Lou, soaring eastward across the Nevada desert, cruise control set, convertible top down, CD player up full-blast, singing "Come Fly With Me" at the top of our lungs.

We were headed back to Madison, a novice cancer survivor and his future-superstar daughter, just days away from completing the magnificent journey which occupied almost three months of my life and five weeks of hers.

We logged over seven thousand miles - more than five thousand with the top down. We swam in the ocean and cool mountain lakes, tanned in the hot desert sun. We got to know big flashy cities and languid little towns. We made many new friends and became even better friends with each other.

And, in what was the main purpose of the trip, but later seemed almost like an incidental bonus, I was successfully treated for prostate cancer at Loma Linda University Medical Center.

To say we had turned something bad into something good would be an understatement.

I had slammed the door on a demon and opened the gate to an incredible journey she and I would never forget.

This is the story of that journey.

Chapter One

My hopes were high that late January day, as I pulled into the medical center parking lot in Madison. It was a couple of weeks before the groundhog would see his shadow and scurry back inside to contemplate the quarterly delusion the natives of Wisconsin call the "change of season."

I was returning to see Dr. Frank Kilpatrick, my longtime "primary physician," who had told me three months earlier that my liver readings were elevated. I had just completed a self-imposed ninety-day low carb diet, during which I exercised daily, and abstained from any alcohol. It was a purposeful effort to avoid having to endure an intrusive liver biopsy. And, more importantly, to preserve my health.

When I walked into the doctor's office thirty pounds lighter, I was feeling great. I seemed to be in perfect health, and was enjoying success at my new business of web site design and marketing.

I'd made a break from the vexatious world of corporate management just two years earlier, leaving my job as Executive Vice-President and General Manager of five Madison radio stations to become my own boss. Life was good!

Then Dr. Kilpatrick said, "Your liver tests are normal, but your PSA score is over seven. I'm referring you to a urologist." I didn't have a clue.

From my radio days, a PSA was a Public Service Announcement. In this case PSA meant Prostate Specific Antigen. Later I learned that a score of anything over four is cause for alarm.

Then on February 12th, after performing a biopsy, Dr. Andrew Graf, the urologist, announced,"You have prostate cancer and it appears to be at an aggressive stage. Your Gleason score is eight on a scale of ten."

Huh? Gleason score? I thought that was a TV rating from the Fifties.

"A Gleason score of eight means the cancer is at a stage where it will grow rapidly. I recommend surgery; that's the gold standard," the doctor said. Then he described the procedure and briefly explained some other options. He told me to think it over and emphasized that I should not take too long to decide.

I didn't idle at the intersection of *Why Me and To Hell with This* for long, nor did I go "into denial" as tradition would have it. I knew what I was faced with. Cancer gremlins were chattering and in the distance I could hear some *big dogs* barking.

Big dogs can scare you with a snarl; frighten you by their stance, invade your imagination. They intimidate you just because they know they *can*.

A bull was loose. I was enraged that these creatures had invaded my being; I but did not waste time recoiling in fear or becoming absorbed in anger. I grabbed the bull by the horns, and set out to learn as much as I could about the disease and how best to deal with it.

While I highly respect Dr. Graf and his abilities as a urologist and surgeon, I wanted to find out what alternatives existed. Within ten days, and with the help of many web sites and several books, I educated myself about the disease and various forms of treatment. I learned that there were differing opinions about which treatment is best. Surgeons recommended surgery. Radiologists recommended radiology. Some doctors suggested radiation seed implants or cryosurgery.

Upon searching further, I learned of a precise form of advanced radiation treatment which involves protons.

Following extensive research and an immense amount of soul-searching, I believe my most important conclusion was:

After a man has seriously studied the options, he must decide what's best for him. Once he has done that, and has committed to his decision, he will find visits by the imaginary cancer gremlins will go away and the *big dogs* will quiet down.

For me the choice was proton radiation treatment, then available only at Loma Linda University Medical Center in Southern California, at the Northeast Proton Treatment Center at Massachusetts General Hospital in Boston, and at Indiana University in Bloomington.

Loma Linda is where proton radiation was first used in a hospital-based treatment facility, in 1990, and it is where the most prostate cancer patients have been treated by this method.

After visiting several websites, exchanging emails and having phone conversations with former patients, I called Loma Linda to determine if I could get the treatment within a reasonable length of time. I wondered about a waiting list. I was transferred to Nurse Sharon Hoyle, right-hand angel to Dr. Carl Rossi.

She asked me if I could forward my lab reports and doctors' consultation records to Dr. Rossi for review. I assured her I could.

I called the medical center in Madison and asked how soon I could get copies of the relevant documents. I picked them up the next afternoon and called Sharon Hoyle to confirm the mailing address at Loma Linda, so I could send the records by the fastest express available.

Unfamiliar with medical personnel being readily accessible, I was surprised to hear nurse Hoyle ask, "Do you have a fax machine? Good. Send the reports. Dr. Rossi's here."

Twenty minutes later she called back and said, "Dr. Rossi says you are a good candidate for proton treatment. He'd like you to schedule a pelvic MRI and a consultation with him."

Checking with the urologist, Dr. Graf, I learned that an MRI of the type Dr. Rossi had requested was a test they had just recently introduced in Madison, and yes, they could do it. But, there was a waiting list.

I decided to find out if I could have it done sooner at Loma Linda and meet with Dr. Rossi as part of the same trip.

Nurse Hoyle was able to schedule the MRI to be performed Monday, March 1st, and I was to meet with the doctor three days later.

I logged on to the Internet and booked a round-trip flight to Ontario, California, the major air-port nearest Loma Linda.

As I clicked "purchase ticket" and hit the *enter* key on my keyboard, I looked up at the small, slightly faded photo that hung on my office wall.

It was me, at age nine, posing with my arm around a Great Dane who was almost as tall as me. My mother had taken the picture while we were on a vacation trip in New England around 1950. At some stop along the way, in Connecti-cut I believe, we met up with this friendly giant.

Though I had never seen him before, I went right up to him and confidently put my arm across his broad shoulders.

My mom snapped the picture which, more than

fifty years later, would still hang in my office, with the inscription:

"Don't Fear the Big Dogs–Billy Vancil, Age 9."

Chapter Two

The sometimes permeating smog was hardly noticeable, on that Leap Day, Sunday, February 29th, as I felt the reassuring jostle of rubber touching concrete on the runway at Ontario.

While driving the twenty-five minutes to Loma Linda in my gray Hyundai rental car, I sensed that this was the start of an experience that would be not only life-saving, but life changing.

The mountains sixty miles east of Los Angeles were still covered with clean white snow, but the sun was warm and the sky was bright blue with hope. The Wisconsin chill in my bones began to evaporate and with it, the fear I'd secretly held within.

Before leaving Madison, I had reserved a room at the Hilton in San Bernardino, the big brawny neighbor of the more genteel Loma Linda. The hotel was across the street from a Mexican restaurant called, "Guadala Harry's." Loma Linda University Medical Center was just ten minutes away from the Hilton but worlds apart from any other place I'd ever been.

I drove around exploring the medical campus the same night I arrived. My appointment for the pelvic MRI was scheduled for seven A.M. and I wanted to find out the night before where I would be going for this high-tech exam.

Thanks to my advance reconnaissance, I arrived for my appointment twenty minutes early the next morning. I had to wait for the first-arriving employee to unlock the door before I could enter the building. The test went smoothly and the technician told me he would be forwarding the results to Dr. Rossi in time for my consultation on Thursday, March 4th.

The next couple of days I lived out of my suitcase, doing a bit of sightseeing, getting lost a couple of times and watching the NCAA basketball tourney on TV, but mainly waiting anxiously for my meeting with Dr. Rossi.

Thursday arrived and I met Dr. Carl Rossi for the first time. He appeared younger than I'd pictured him. I felt comfortable in his presence as he explained how he would use a series of highly focused proton beams to precisely deliver the correct dosage into my body at various angles, in order to treat the cancer without damaging surrounding tissue. That is something that cannot be done with traditional, less precise radiation delivery.

He said I should go back to Wisconsin, take a drug called Casodex and have Lupron shots (a man-made hormone that slows the growth of cancer and makes treatment more effective).

After being on Casodex and Lupron for two months I was to return to Loma Linda, around May 15th, to begin proton radiation treatment.

Long before making the trip to California for this preliminary consultation, I was so certain of my decision that I had already sought and found a place to stay in Loma Linda during the time I would be there for treatment. I knew that staying at the Hilton for nearly three months would be both out of budget and out of character for me, so I had called Nurse Sharon Hoyle for advice.

She recommended a particular duplex she thought I would like and suggested I call the owner right away to see if it was available. I was delighted to find it was not yet booked for early May through early August.

I was told the place had two bedrooms, two baths, kitchen, living room, office, and a large deck with a mountain view. And, it was within walking distance of the medical center. High speed internet connection and unlimited long distance phone service were included in the rent. I mailed the security deposit as soon as I hung up the phone.

Never one to buy things sight unseen, I told Lorraine, the owner, "Now, while I'm there for my preliminary meeting I will drive past, and if I see any ghosts peeking out, can I change my mind?" It was my polite way of saying, "If I don't like the looks of the place, can I back out?"

In the charitable manner so common in Loma Linda she said, "Of course; we want you to be comfortable. But I don't think you'll see any ghosts peeking out."

My future home away from home, on San Lucas Drive, featured palm trees and conifers side-by- side, mockingbirds singing, geckos scurrying. The round, white towers of compassionate Loma Linda Medical Center majestically guarded the neighborhood.

With the snow-covered San Bernardino Mountains standing proudly in the background, a myriad of tree types, including the tallest palm trees I'd ever seen, populated the landscape.

The place was beautiful! I couldn't wait to see the view from the deck; and if there were ghosts, they would have to wait a couple of months.

After consuming two soft tacos and a tall iced tea at Guadala Harry's, I headed for the rental car return center in Ontario. It was there, on the shuttle between the rental company office and the airport that a significant moment occurred.

The driver of the shuttle had unloaded some people who had come from the airport to pick up their rental cars. I asked him if there'd be a wait to return, since I was the only passenger in sight at the moment.

He said, "It's slow today. Hop in. Let's go."

I loaded my baggage onto the bus and we took off for the terminal; just the two of us on board. The driver looked to be about my age, perhaps a few years younger. He asked what brought me to California. I told him that I had been meeting with doctors at Loma Linda University and would be returning in a couple of months to start proton radiation treatment. He seemed moderately interested, pretended to know about Loma Linda, and seemed willing to chat.

Thinking he could care less, I continued the discourse, "The last time I was in California for a couple of months was when I took Advanced Infantry Training at Fort Ord, just outside San Francisco."

"Really," he said, "When were you there?"

"It was March and April of 1967. Almost forty years ago," I told him.

"How about that?" he said, "so was I."

Surprised, I said, "Before that, in January and February, I was in Basic Training at Fort Lewis, Washington."

"So was I," said the driver, "We were there at the same time. Remember how it rained almost every day?"

"Have you had your prostate checked lately?" I blurted out.

"You know, as you were talking about Loma Linda and this proton treatment," he replied pensively, "I was thinking I should have that PSA test done soon. I can't remember *ever* having it checked."

"I think you should," I said seriously. Then I asked, "Does this happen often, just having one passenger on the shuttle?"

"Very seldom." He smiled.

"It must have happened today for a reason," I said as I headed for the terminal and handed him two dollars for unloading my baggage.

"Don't forget; tell your doctor you want a PSA test," I added sternly.

"Thanks for the tip," he said, as he got back on the bus; putting the vehicle in gear, with a smile and what sounded like a sigh of relief.

I knew when he thanked me for the "tip"; it wasn't the two dollars he was referring to. That's when I began to believe something had led me to the web page where I first learned of Loma Linda. I was there for a reason.

And, something had put me on the shuttle that day, alone with my Viet Nam-era boot camp comrade, who accepted one more command.

It was the first of several "I must have been there for a reason" moments that I would experience during and after the remarkable journey.

Chapter Three

It was now March 5th and I was back in Madison, relieved to tell everyone that the MRI test performed at Loma Linda showed no signs of the disease having spread and that I was scheduled to start proton therapy in two months. May 18th was the designated start date for my treatments.

It was time to prepare for the trip which would put me in California for a three month stay. I would be making this first leg of the journey alone. Tori Lou would fly out to join me after school let out for the summer. I'd never been away for that long before. What to pack? What not to pack? Who would take care of my cat, Charli, and water my plants? How will we get everything in the car? My unflappable Tori Lou would help figure it out.

Luckily, the web design and internet-related work I was doing could be done from anywhere, so keeping up with my business was not a problem. I'd just pack up the computers, some file folders and sticky notes; and plug into the web when I got there. Most of my clients wouldn't even know I was gone, and those who did wouldn't care, as long as I stayed connected.

I was enthusiastic about the upcoming trip, but my spirits were suddenly dampened when I received a letter stating that the insurance company was sorry, but they would not be able to cover the proton radiation treatment. They said it was "experimental," in their opinion. I guess I should have expected a roadblock of some sort to pop up. But, this?

We were talking many tens of thousands of dollars! Suddenly, I was standing at the inter-section of *It's a Wonderful World* and *There Goes My Everything*.

With help from a longtime attorney friend, Jerry McAdow, himself a prostate cancer survi-vor, I started compiling documentation which we thought would prove the validity of proton radiation treatment. We hoped to convince the insurance company to reverse their decision. The process became more time-consuming and tedious than I ever would have imagined.

"I'm just as determined to win this battle with the insurance company as I am to win the bat-tle with cancer," I told Jerry. "And, I'm not sure which is going to be more difficult."

One thing was for sure. Regardless of whether the insurance company ultimately decided to pay, I was going ahead with my plan. I told the comptrollers at Loma Linda that I would be personally responsible for any payment not covered by insurance. I wasn't sure how I would handle the huge expense, but I had to believe that somehow I would figure out a way.

With the unsettled issue of insurance on the back burner, I continued my preparations and the date of departure snuck up on me very quickly. All of a sudden, it was time to go.

Tori Lou's mother, Laura, and I had divorced several years before, but we remained good friends, shared important moments in the life of Victoria Louise (legal term for Tori Lou) and lived only a few miles apart. During the couple of weeks prior to my departure, Tori Lou had been staying with me to offer sage advice as I prepared for the trip.

With Tori Lou's help, I had effectively packed all I needed (and more) into the car and was ready to depart for California. I returned Tori Lou to the safekeeping of her mom on Mother's Day, May 9th.

That Sunday morning saying goodbye to "Lou" (as I call her sometimes) was tough, even though I knew she would be joining me in Loma Linda in a couple of months.

"It's OK, Dad. We can talk over the Internet and on the phone," she assured me.

"I know. Now, listen to your mom, okay? And, finish strong these last couple weeks in school, okay? Don't forget to brush Charli. And, don't get hurt. You can't learn to surf if you're on crutches," I stalled.

We were both crying by the time I finally got in the car and drove off slowly. I watched in the rearview mirror as Lou forced a smile and waved goodbye until I was out of sight.

With the cruise control set, I piled up the miles. The hum of the highway was hypnotic and comforting. Once the sobbing stopped part way into Iowa, I began contemplating what it all meant.

I was at peace with the decision I had made, despite not yet seeing a thumbs up from the insurance company.

Because I had studied all the options so carefully and received so much positive input from the doctors at Loma Linda, I had complete confidence that I would return home healthy and wise–wealthy didn't matter.

Chapter Four

I drove all the way to Lexington, Nebraska the first night. As I squinted through the darkness looking for a motel sign, there were thunderstorms off to both the north and the south, tossing out lightning bolts like a Vegas blackjack dealer flipping fives.

The next morning, watching the Weather Channel, I learned there were tornadoes in that deck of storms. It was the last rain I would even come close to for almost three months.

Just before I found my safe haven half way across the Cornhusker State, my cell phone had rung. It was Tori Lou! What a surprise!

"Hi, Lou. Yeah, I'm okay. Almost got caught in a storm! But, I'm okay. And, I'm looking for a motel with *color* TV!" I joked.

When I was a kid traveling with my folks, I always wanted to stop at a place with TV, shuffleboard or best of all, a swimming pool.

"Hey, Dad. Are you anywhere near Grand Island?" Tori Lou asked with a curious confidence.

"Yeah, I saw a sign for it a ways back. How'd you know?" I answered, so glad to hear her voice.

"Well, you left at ten-thirty this morning and Mom and I thought you'd be averaging about sixty-five, so I tracked you on the map," she explained.

Wow! What a kid. I slept well that night, knowing that Tori Lou had things well under control back home.

The storms played themselves out in the night, and I had clear sailing the next day, finishing off Nebraska and taking on Colorado. As the Rocky Mountains started to come into view in the distance, it reminded me again of the trips I had enjoyed as a kid with my mom and step-father. I will never forget seeing the Rockies on the horizon the first time, nor this time.

My mind flashed back to the mid-50s, when I was about Tori Lou's age. My travels with Frank and Minnie were legendary back in Kewanee, Illinois. One summer we went to Europe and I showed slides to the Lions Club when we came back. Businessmen in Kewanee were easily entertained in those days.

Before I finished high school, I'd been to forty-eight states and twelve foreign countries, without ever going on an airplane. My step-father, Frank, would not fly; so all our traveling was done by car, train, bus or boat.

The experience I gained from those travels was, as the credit card commercial says, "priceless." That's one of the reasons I was looking forward to the return trip from California to Wisconsin with Tori Lou as my co-pilot.

But, for now it was just me, the Interstate and my unlikely collection of CDs which included Michael Buble, The Temptations, Hootie & the Blowfish, UB40 and Connie Francis singing Italian songs in German.

By lunch time the second day out, I'd made it to Denver and the weather was great. I drove through the mountains with the top down, even though snow had closed the roads in that area, just two weeks before.

I stopped and asked a truck driver to take my picture at a "scenic view" area 10,000 feet up. I saw Vail without snow, went through Glenwood Springs, home of the largest hot springs pool in the world, stopped to stretch in a place called Parachute, crossed the Colorado River about eight times, and drove through some seemingly endless tunnels before the Rockies released me from their spell. It was starting to get dark when I got to Grand Junction, Colorado, elevation 4,586. Although I was energized by the drive through the mountains and could have kept going, something told me to stop and get my bearings.

At the far edge of the city, I noticed a truck stop with about twenty semi-trailer trucks parked in a row. They were spaced so evenly and at just the right diagonal that you could tell they'd done this before. Something told me this might just be the edge of the world. I pulled in next to the big rigs, my Mitsubishi Spyder looking like a little silver gnat next to the massive eighteen-wheelers. I spotted a couple of drivers, toothpicks active, coming out of the restaurant.

In my best "good buddy" voice I asked, "Can you guys tell me what's on down the road from here?"

"For about two-hundred and ten miles—nothing!" one of them said, as he relocated his toothpick to the opposite corner of his mouth with an incurious twist of the tongue.

So, it *is* the edge of the world. I was right.

"Seems like a good place to stop for the night," I replied, and then went back onto the Interstate and checked into a motel that I'd passed earlier.

About six-thirty the next morning, I gassed up the car; bought some pure Rocky Mountain bottled water and some Juicy Fruit gum and set off across the Utah desert. The truck drivers were correct. There was nothing, except majestic mesas and towering buttes, for more than two-hundred miles.

For a place that was always ominous and could be threatening at times, the desert seemed somehow trying to offer entertainment, if not comfort, as it whipped up little sand devils - then made them dance away.

I saw a lone antelope standing in the middle of sand-packed nothingness. What was he doing there? He may have been thinking the same about me. I wondered if antelopes ever get cancer. Probably not.

Once Utah was in my rearview mirror, I clipped the corner of Arizona and then found myself in Nevada. It was Tuesday, May 11th and I thought, "Wow, I'm going to make five states in one day and without ever getting on a plane."

"What happens in Las Vegas stays in Las Vegas," the ad campaign had proclaimed. Well, I didn't stop, so nothing really happened that I would want to leave there. But, even though I didn't wager at any casinos, I was about to take a different kind of risk: driving Interstate 15 from Las Vegas to San Bernardino!

In Southern California, it's not uncommon to hear people say, "The biggest gamble in going to Las Vegas is the drive there and back."

After several stop-and-go hours in construction zones and way too many inhalations of second-hand diesel smoke, I completed the survival course offered by the I-15, and finally saw the green sign that said "Loma Linda University Next Exit."

As I pulled out of the fast lane onto Waterman Avenue, the sun was just starting to descend behind Mount Baldy.

Old Sol seemed to sigh with relief as he settled in behind the mountains for the night. The exhausting assignment of watching over my driving was almost done for the day.

I'd traveled one thousand, nine-hundred and sixty-three miles since I had hugged Tori Lou goodbye, hardly thirty hours earlier. It seemed as though a year had passed.

I recognized the campus neighborhood from my previous visit, back in March, and I headed straight for San Lucas Drive.

Chapter Five

Somewhere, part way through Utah, I had learned via cell phone from Jerry McAdow that some progress had been made with my insurance company. They had agreed to the extent that they would consider paying a portion of the cost of proton treatment, but only if I underwent laparoscopic surgery first, to find out if the cancer had spread into my pelvic lymph nodes.

Okay, now let's think about this. I drove two thousand miles to avoid surgery; now they want me to have surgery. Laparoscopic surgery? What's that?

"Well," Dr. Rossi said thoughtfully, when I told him about this on the phone, "It's a relatively minor procedure and it would give us some valuable information upon which to base the treatment plan. Why not, if the insurance company will pay for it? We'll just start your proton treatments two weeks after the surgery. That'll give you a chance to recuperate."

Recuperate? From a *minor* procedure? Finally, I came to accept the fact that it was a good idea for the doctors to see just what was in there, or more importantly *not* in there, and plan my treatment accordingly.

"After all, they're not cutting me wide open," I rationalized. "Just a couple of tiny holes to put in a tiny camera and have a look around, take a few little samples." Still, I was not able to classify it as minor. I preferred to rank it as minor *elevated.*

I was too tired from driving all day to worry any more about it right then, and besides, I was almost "home." I had no trouble finding the place on San Lucas Drive that I'd driven by so many times two months earlier. There it was!

I had called the landlord, Lorraine, from my cell phone and she was waiting with the key. Inside, I found large rooms, beautifully and totally furnished - and not a single ghost.

It wasn't easy to sleep that first night, though the bed was comfortable and the place seemed like home right from the start. I knew that this was just the beginning; there was much to do, much to anticipate. What about this surgery thing?

And, what will the insurance company do?

In the next couple of days I would have some preliminary lab tests, attend my first support group meeting at the medical center and meet with Dr. Baldwin, the surgeon who would be putting the camera inside me for that procedure I'd tagged, "minor elevated."

On the day after my arrival, I went to my first support group meeting at the medical center.

About eighty people were sitting at long tables eating small triangular egg salad sandwiches along with macadamia nut cookies and their choice of some nondescript fruit juice or water.

"Are there any returning alumni here tonight?" Gerry Troy opened the meeting, to find out how many former proton radiation patients were there.

Six or seven hands went up. There was a doctor named Roy from Vermont, who returns every six months because he loves Loma Linda and the nearby desert; Chuck from Pennsylvania, who played 730 holes of golf during his treatment and was feeling fine. He, along with John from Florida, had returned to play in the Proton Golf Tournament, which has raised over two million dollars for the Ken Venturi Cancer Research Chair.

Another alumnus, Dr. Arnd Hallmeyer, an MD from Berlin, Germany was there to report that he was doing fine and had reduced his PSA score from an unfathomable 436 to 0.1.

Also attending was Bob Marckini from Massachusetts, founder of the Brotherhood of the Balloon, an international prostate cancer support group. It's a fraternity of former proton patients who stay in touch through an online newsletter, website (www.protonbob.com) and reunions.

The Brotherhood, at that time, numbered more than 1,500 members.

While it was called a support group meeting, I saw no one there who appeared to be in need of much support. In fact, as I mentioned to some people I met that night, "I've never seen so many old men with smiles on their faces since the Ho-Chunk Nation opened a bingo hall in Madison a few years ago."

They told jokes, served refreshments, exchanged stories and, to a person, had high praise for Loma Linda and the treatment they had received. I wished that somebody from the insurance company could have been there.

Loma Linda University Medical Center, celebrating its 100th Anniversary in 2005, had been doing proton radiation treatments for nearly 15 years with a success rate as good as any form of prostate cancer treatment. This was about as experimental as the waffle iron.

One of the conditions, regarding the insurance company's willingness to pay for my proton treatment, was that the results of the surgery had to be negative. There must be no evidence of spreading of the cancer, if they were going to pay anything.

I was pretty confident the surgery would produce the hoped-for outcome. After all, I had already had a cat scan, a bone scan, and an ultrasound back in Madison, a pelvic MRI in Loma Linda, and several other tests I couldn't remember.

But, nonetheless, I was starting to second guess my decision about having the laparoscopic surgery.

I thought, "Maybe I should just try to figure out some way to pay for this over time. I know what the outcome of the surgery's going to be. I came here to *not* have surgery."

I called my trusted friend and attorney, Jerry, and he helped me think it through more clearly.

"You've got the best of both," he assured me with cautious confidence. "The minor surgery will provide valuable information that will give you confidence as you start the proton treatment.

It's perfect. And, the insurance company will pay for it–I think."

I didn't like the "I think" part, but I knew he was right. "Okay, let's go for it," I decided. "If I chicken out now, I will never know for sure if the cancer has spread," I convinced myself.

Now that I had that settled, I wanted to get to know this place, called Southern California, a little better. It was May 15th and the weather continued to be perfect–sunshine, mid 80's and low humidity.

That first weekend in Loma Linda, I stayed in my comfort zone of fifteen miles or so, as I scrutinized the landscape.

I found the post office, car wash, supermarkets, workout center, about twelve Mexican restaurants, and located the nearest ATM machine - plus a backup one just in case I emptied out the first one.

I'd made it a point to look for skateboard shops and skate parks in the area. I knew this would be of major interest to Tori Lou when she arrived. Over the past year or so she had become an avid skateboarder. On May 1st, shortly before I left Madison for Loma Linda, she had placed second in a skateboard competition which featured a field of eleven contestants–all boys, but her.

In Redlands, I found a skate shop called Icon and one of the guys in the store told me the closest skate park was about ten minutes away in Yucaipa. "Just get on The Ten (Interstate 10) and watch for the Yucaipa exit. Take a left and go about a mile. It's kind of out in the middle of nowhere," he explained. "Turn left on the road that's straight across from Farmer Boy's."

It looked like a nice skate park, and the sign across the street at Farmer Boy's said, "Best Hamburger in the World." How could I be so lucky? Who would have thought that I would find the world's best burger here in this place; in the middle of nowhere, yet also in the middle of everything in southern California?

Yucaipa, Loma Linda, Redlands, and San Bernardino are all located in the part of California that is called the Inland Empire. It's just an hour from the Pacific beaches, an hour from Palm Springs, two hours from San Diego and just over an hour from Los Angeles. In the winter, it's possible to snowboard in the nearby mountains and surf where the Beach Boys grew up, all in the same day.

Every time I heard, "Let's go surfin' now . . ." coming out of the ceiling of one of the Stater Brothers' Supermarkets, I was reminded of one of my favorite old radio memories. It was the early Sixties and the Beach Boys' song *Barbara Ann* was high on the charts. The group had performed at the Masonic Temple in Davenport, Iowa where I was program director at the popular top forty AM station, KSTT.

I was the emcee for the concert and, afterwards, I talked the Beach Boys into coming to the studios to record some promos for the station. There they were: Brian, Dennis, Mike and Al, not yet so famous they wouldn't honor a young disk jockey by riding in his '54 Chevy.

Having concluded my weekend of touring Yucaipa and several adjoining communities, I was pulling into the carport at the duplex Sunday evening, when I saw a neighbor across the alley walking a St. Bernard. Being a big fan of big dogs, I went over and introduced myself. I learned that the dog's name was Sebastian.

His owner, Noreen, said that he was very friendly and loved to go for walks. I told Noreen that my daughter loved Saint Bernards and that Tori Lou and Sebastian would have to meet.

"Just have Tori Lou come over when she gets here," said Noreen, "and if she wants, she can take Sebastian for a walk. He'd love that."

When I talked to Tori Lou that night on the phone I told her about Sebastian, and she could hardly wait to meet him.

"Hey, I've got one new friend in Loma Linda and I'm not even there yet," she said, as we signed off for the night.

Chapter Six

Monday, May 17th, I was prepped for my proton treatment and underwent some pre-op for the surgery as well. In preparation for the proton treatments, they had me lie down in a half-pipe of PVC material with a plastic sheet under my body and poured some warm, gooey foam material under the sheet. The stuff hardened in a few minutes creating a "mold" of my body. This was my "pod," the magical vehicle I would ride to wellness. Before my treatment was completed about two months later, I would have climbed in and out of this unorthodox, but effective, contraption forty-four times.

A pod, or mold, is created for each patient to immobilize him while the proton beam silently and painlessly enters the prostate area and does battle with the cancer cells.

Having completed this advance work for the proton radiation therapy, there was still the matter of the minor surgical procedure. To prep for that I went to another part of the hospital and received an electrocardiogram, a chest x-ray, about a half dozen blood tests, and was given instructions to not eat anything after midnight. The laparoscopic surgery was scheduled for very early the next morning. I was told to be at the pre-op room at 5:30 A.M.

Even though I was going into surgery the next day, I had to keep up with my work. One of the activities I had continued by long distance was a couponing web site, *MadisonCoupons.com.* I had created this web-based business a couple of years earlier and it had an advertiser base of about fifty clients. Periodically, I sent a mass email out to a database of persons who'd signed up to receive updates. I called this group the Coupon Club. To make the emails more interesting I included a trivia question at the end of each message.

That evening after all the prep work at the hospital was completed; I was preparing to send out one of the coupon updates, and trying to think up a good trivia question. The duplex I was renting featured a large well-stocked bookcase in the room I was using as my office. I decided to look through the collection to get an idea for a trivia question. One of the books was Lawrence Welk's biography, *Wunnerful, Wunnerful.*

When I opened it, I saw it was autographed by Lawrence himself! Impressive, but I didn't find a good trivia question within the pages of his life story.

So much for the idea of quickly finding my trivia question in a book. Because I was in a hurry, I relied on the method I most often used in searching for trivia. I called up the search engine Google on the computer. I'd learned that typing "This Day in History" almost always yielded usable trivia material; so I started with that. The first thing that came up was a page from the History Channel web site that said, "On this date in 1992, Lawrence Welk died in Santa Monica, California." Yikes! There *were* ghosts in this place after all! At least in the computer. A one and a two . . . turn off the bubble machine.

The next day, Tuesday, May 18th, was the date my proton treatment was to have begun. But, because of the insurance company's insistence on my having the laparoscopic surgery, I was headed for the operating room instead.

It was still dark that morning when I walked from my duplex across the parking lot of the Loma Linda University School of Nursing, across the emergency room driveway, into the almost deserted hallway to the elevator that would take me to the seventh floor.

As I checked in, the nurse at the reception desk computer asked me the usual sign-in questions, and then asked, "Where did you park your car, or did someone drop you off here?"

"Actually, I walked here," I said.

"And, you live in Wisconsin?" she asked.

"Yes," I said. "But, I didn't walk from Wisconsin. I have a place a couple of blocks from here that I'm renting."

"I see," the nurse smiled, "It's just that we don't have too many patients walk in for their surgery. You will be in the pre-op room for awhile before surgery and we'll have the doctors and nurses come in to get you ready. If you have any questions, don't be afraid to ask them."

The only question that came to mind was, "If this turns out the way I hope, will the insurance company pay for all of my treatment?" But, I knew they would not be able to answer that one. I would just have to go under anesthesia not knowing.

I told myself, "It's going to be okay. You will find out soon enough and the answer will be good." A nurse came in and gave me a shot.

"This will make you drowsy," she told me.

The next thing I knew, a fuzzy picture of "later that day" was coming into view and I had a pain in my gut that was definitely more than minor.

When I came to, a nurse told me that they wanted me to walk as soon as possible to prevent clotting. Walk? I could hardly lift my knee! Walking would have to wait awhile.

Then Doctor Baldwin came in and told me that the surgery took almost four hours and eleven samples of lymph nodes were taken. He said that the nodes which were examined during the operation, showed no cancer.

However, some of the samples had been sent off to a lab and it might be as much as three days until I found out about those.

I knew it was going to be a long three days, waiting for those results. The clock on the wall in my room was the slowest moving timepiece I'd ever seen. To my surprise, much sooner than I expected him to, Dr. Baldwin walked into the room with a clip board and a big smile.

The news had arrived early.

"Usually we don't get these results back this soon," the doctor told me, "but I guess the lab must not be very busy right now; we just received the report and they found no cancer in any of the sample lymph nodes."

This good news meant the plan for the proton radiation treatment could be calculated more precisely and would not have to be augmented by standard radiation, the kind which can cause adverse side effects. This "minor procedure" had produced major information! And it would turn out to be significant in our discussions with the insurance company.

A swell of relief overcame any pain I was feeling as I took the doctor's hand and thanked him for what he'd done.

The next couple of days consisted of sleeping, watching the Travel Channel, walking the hospital hallways, sleeping, watching some other channels, walking around, trying to eat nondescript hospital food, sleeping, walking around some more, and then repeating the process.

Those seventy-two hours, or so, remain a blur because of the pain medication, but I'll always remember being stuck in the hospital bed and watching the clock that hardly moved.

Chapter Seven

It was Friday, May 21st, and I was back "home" at the rental unit on San Lucas recovering from the surgery. I was anxious for the proton radiation treatments to start. Each day, I felt a little less pain from the surgery and I moved around a little better. When the time came to climb into the pod, I would be ready. For the next several days I laid low, letting my body heal and keeping up with my work using the internet and long distance phone.

I was feeling more and more at home in this place called Loma Linda, but other than Dr. Rossi, Dr. Baldwin, Nurse Sharon Hoyle, my landlord Lorraine, Noreen and Sebastian, I had not yet become acquainted with anyone else. There were a few fellow patients I met casually in the hospital and at the first support group meeting, but no one I could actually call a new friend. That was about to change.

On Wednesday, May 26th, I was trying to decide if I should go to the support group meeting that night. It had been a week since my surgery and I was feeling pretty good. There was a knock at the door. I peeked through the fisheye hole in the door and saw a tall guy in khaki pants and a crisp, long-sleeved, white shirt.

"He's not holding a pizza or flowers; I wonder who he is," I thought, as I opened the door.

"How y'all doin,'" he drawled, "I'm your dahnstairs neighbor, Robert McDaniel."

"Hi, Robert. I'm Bill, from Wisconsin," I answered.

"Well, we just wanted to let you know we're in the unit downstairs, my wife Martha and I, if you ever need anything," explained this easy-going long tall Texan from Abilene. "That's our big ol' tank out back there. I had to park at an angle it's so long." I had noticed the bright red, super-sized Ford Excursion with Texas plates before, and thought, "Now that would be a lot easier to pack than a convertible."

Robert was a proton patient who'd arrived about a week before I had. He's a car collector with about twenty-five cars, ranging from 1900s to late-1950s models, in his collection back in Abilene. The old car books he'd bought at some flea markets would later become a fascination of Tori Lou's.

From reading those books, talking with Robert and looking at pictures of his car collection, she became a young fan of automobilia.

And, what a great place for old car watching–
Southern California!

Robert's wife, Martha, also did a kind of work
she could take along with her, doing some lit-
erary editing on her computer during their
stay. They both loved making the rounds of
various supermarkets and restaurants and
started giving me some shopping and dining
tips.

Over the next few weeks, they would become
good friends to me and later to Tori Lou as
well.

One of the most prized things Tori Lou and I
would later take home was a standing invitation to visit the McDaniels in Abilene.

Chapter Eight

It was Memorial Day - Monday, May 31, 2004. My proton treatments were to start the next day. In Southern California they have an annual phenomenon they call "June Gloom."

Unusually heavy coastal fog occurs around this time of year and combines with smog drifting over from Los Angeles, causing the view of the mountains to be obscured part of the day and the sunshine to lose some of its brilliance.

This is Southern California's version of the change of seasons. It's less extreme than Wisconsin's, where the leaves fall off the trees, the temperature drops dozens of degrees, the ground gets covered with white stuff and the checkout clerks at the supermarket become less personable.

I decided to spend Memorial Day just exploring, relaxing and enjoying the weather. I drove into San Bernadino, past Guadala Harry's and the Hilton, where I had stayed back in March.

I turned North on Waterman, which becomes Highway 18, a four-lane wandering climb up the mountain toward what's known as the "Rim of the World." I drove for about half an hour, and found myself at an altitude of a couple of thousand feet higher and felt a cooler temperature. The view was magnificent. I vowed this was a place I would visit again and, next time, I would go further up the mountain.

As I was returning from my brief excursion, I passed Montecito Memorial Park, a beautiful cemetery on Barton Road at the edge of Loma Linda. On this Memorial Day, the place was filled with colorful gravesite displays of flowers, balloons and shiny pinwheels.

The region has a large Latino population and the Latinos are lavish and festive in their remembrances. It was indeed a day to remember and to celebrate life. Before falling asleep that night, I made a mental note to write a poem someday that might begin with the line, "Where birds sing at night, and angels pose as nurses dressed in blue . . ."

The next day, my treatments would begin, and it would be "one down and forty-three to go." I slept well, thankful for where I was and all I had experienced so far.

Chapter Nine

My first treatment on June 1st was scheduled for 9:20 A.M. Later I found out that most first-timers go in at that about that time. The first treatment takes a few minutes longer, because of the initial setup required with the pod and computers, so that time is reserved for patients climbing into their pod for the first treatment.

The procedure went as though it had been rehearsed many times. In fact, for the technicians running the show, it had not only been rehearsed, but performed countless times. For me, it had only been rehearsed in my mind.

As a patient described it at one of the support meetings, "They get you all lined up in your pod, check the computers, reassure you that everything's okay, you won't feel a thing, and then they all run out of the room."

After some whirring and beeping sounds, the technicians come back. The patient gets out of the pod, not having felt a thing, and goes off to do whatever he wants to do with the rest of his day. It sounds simple, but it took four decades, for physicists, engineers, and physicians from around the world, working together, to develop proton radiation treatment.

It first became available at Loma Linda in 1990 and thousands of patients have received proton treatment at the University Medical Center since then.

I learned that after the first treatment, any new guy gets bounced around in the schedule for the first couple of weeks and eventually settles into a daily routine. I hoped to have a time of around eight-thirty A.M. locked in by the time Tori Lou arrived, thinking it would be nice to be able to get up and get the treatment over with and then have the rest of the day to do other things.

Tori Lou agreed and told me over the phone, "Hey, Dad, eighty-thirty would be great if you can get it! You could go get your treatment then come back and wake me up about nine and take me to the beach or a skateboard park! Perfect!" She had it all figured out.

Treatments were scheduled from early morning to late at night every day Monday through Friday. My first couple of appointments were in the evening hours, and then I moved up to late afternoon. I kept dropping hints to Tim, the technician who handled the scheduling, telling him that I wanted "The Morning Show."

Much sooner than I expected, and long before Tori Lou was to arrive, I got my wish. I was only a few days into my treatments when I walked into the gantry and Tim gave me the good news.

"Eight-thirty tomorrow," he told me.

"Great! Can I stay with that time the rest of the way out? You sure? Eight-thirty?" I asked.

"Yep, that'll work," he said.

"What was the Beach Boys last number one hit?" I asked him as I walked away. I had gotten into the habit of asking him a music trivia question every day when I came in. Hey, it's good to be friends with the scheduling guy.

He never got one answer correct, but I guess he thought it was fun anyway, because he would always say, "Oh, yeah. I should've known that."

"*Kokomo,*" I said "You know . . . Aruba, Jamaica, Key Largo . . ."

"Oh, yeah, I should've known that," he smiled.

"Well, do you know who sang the lead on the Beach Boys' hit *Barbara Ann?*"

"I don't know," said Tim, humoring me for the second time in one day.

"Dean Torrance of Jan & Dean," I answered. "Surprised?"

"A little, but I should've known that," Tim shrugged, apparently tired of the game.

During my entire stay in Loma Linda there was no rain. It was the same story every day from weatherman, Johnny Mountain, on the Los Angeles television station, "Sunny and upper-seventies here in your L.A.; cooler at those busy beaches; quite a bit warmer at the Inland Empire and hotter down in the ol' desert."

Generally, "here" means Los Angeles; "the beaches" means Santa Monica, Long Beach, Newport Beach; "inland" means Riverside, San Bernardino, Loma Linda, and the "desert" means Palm Springs.

I had heard reports from back home that in Wisconsin it rained almost every day in May and then in June a tornado hit causing millions of dollars in damage. The very next week, they actually felt an earthquake!

When I heard that, I told a friend on the phone, "Send my stuff. I'm staying here." I said it jokingly, but with a hint of resolve.

There were a few small tremors while I was in Loma Linda. Near the San Andreas Fault little quakes are common, but the news seldom makes better than the lower corner of page three in the San Bernardino Sun.

As I settled into the routine, the days moved by quickly. I managed to stay busy with my work, with two computers hooked up to high-speed Internet connection; plus I'd bought some software that enabled me to connect to and run my computer back in Madison by remote control.

During the week I stayed more or less on Central Daylight Time because most of the people I was working with by email and phone were in either the Midwest or further east. It worked out well for me to get up and start my day around six-thirty A.M., "Eight-thirty Central," as they say on TV.

During the first week in June the discussions back home between my attorney, Jerry

McAdow and the legal counsel for the insurance company had gotten into high gear.

Jerry was maintaining a file of everything and just giving me briefings as it all proceeded. It was a great help to know that he was on top of the situation. It started to appear that they were going to end up paying a sizeable portion, if not all, of the cost of the treatment.

This was good news to receive just when the "June Gloom" was moving in, as Johnny Mountain said it would. The geographical behemoths, named the San Bernardino Mountains (no relation to Johnny) began playing hide-and-seek each morning behind the light brown haze.

It was at least one P.M. each day before one could be assured the mountains were still there.

One of the more interesting work projects I took on by long distance had nothing to do with web site design, but instead put me back to what I did in my early days of radio, announcing.

A company in Madison which builds telephone answering systems had recommended me to record the voice track for a new system they'd built for a home security company. The manager called me.

"Sure, I'd be glad to," I said, "but, I'm in California so I'll have to find a place to record it and I can send it on a CD."

"Can you do that?" the caller asked.

"Sure, piece of cake," I assured him. We agreed on a price and he said he'd email me the scripts. Now, I just had to figure out how to do it.

In the phone book I found Inland Empire Recording Studios in Redlands. I called the owner, Jeff Wilder, and found they'd be happy to rent me studio time and could burn a CD for me. Perfect. I said I would call back once I'd received the scripts.

We left it at that. I'd learned long ago that no job is for sure, until the contract, or in this case, the script, is in hand.

Chapter Ten

It was the morning of June 11th, and I was in Gantry Three, the room where the computerized ninety-ton machine delivered my daily dose of highly targeted radiation. I was climbing in the pod for treatment number nine.

"Who won the Grammy for the Best Rhythm and Blues Recording and three other Grammies in 1960?" I asked Tim.

He responded to my latest trivia question as usual, "I don't know; who?" he asked, as he adjusted my pod to line up properly with the thin red optic laser beams that formed intersecting lines across my sheet-covered chest. These beams were not emitting any radiation; they were just there for the purpose of lining up the "target."

"I'll give you a hint. He died yesterday," I said.

"Oh, Ray Charles. I should have known that," said Tim. "Okay, all set," he added, as he left the room to turn on the machine that would send the positively-charged subatomic particles into my body.

For a few days, watching the local news was like watching national news. Everything seemed to be happening in Southern California right then. Ronald Reagan died in Bel Air. Ray Charles died in Beverly Hills. The Los Angeles Lakers practically died at the Staples Center, in the NBA Finals. Bill Clinton held a book signing in Santa Monica. And, there were a couple of minor earthquakes.

I went on line to the Ronald Reagan Memorial web site and sent an email, knowing Mrs. Reagan would never see it, but it made me feel good to send it.

"Dear Nancy, I admired President Reagan a lot and though we never met, I felt a certain closeness to him, probably because of some similarities in our backgrounds. He was born in Tampico, Illinois, about forty miles from my birthplace, Kewanee. His first full-time radio job was in Davenport, Iowa and so was mine.

And, now so many years later, though I never became a movie star or President, I'm in California not far from Bel Air, where you so compassionately comforted him in his final years.

Thank you, Nancy, for being so good to him. He was a great President."

The next day, I got an email back.

"Thank you. Your kindness and sympathy at this time is of great comfort to Mrs. Reagan."

I printed the page, which showed the Presidential Seal at the top, and added it to my collection of memorabilia.

Chapter Eleven

With some help from the Internet, I'd located several skateboard parks within driving distance of Loma Linda and printed out Map-Quest maps to each of them. I'd found the park at Yucaipa earlier, and had added several more to the list: Van's Skate park at Orange, the historic Upland skate park, a park in Palm Springs, parks at Laguna Niguel and Fontana, and the favorite of many top Orange County skaters - the public skateboard park at Chino.

Tori Lou was so into skateboarding and snow-boarding in Wisconsin that I knew the skate-board parks and beaches would be her favorite places to visit. She had talked about learning to surf from the first moment she found out she was coming to California. I came across a web site for Surf City Surfing Lessons and added it to my "favorites" for future reference.

I completed my fourteenth treatment on the Friday before Father's day. Almost one-third of the way finished with the treatments and everything was going well. Tori Lou called me that Sunday to wish me happy Father's Day.

"I mailed one of your presents, did you get it

yet?" she asked. "I'm bringing the other one with me."

"No, I didn't get it yet, but it will probably arrive tomorrow," I assured her, knowing she probably mailed it the day before, almost forgetting about Father's Day.

"Okay, well the space in my suitcase that I will use to bring your present can be used to put stuff that I buy in California." she explained.

She had overlooked the fact that my present, giving up its space upon presentation to Dad, would then have to go in with Dad's stuff. I was already wondering how we would pack everything when it was time to go home. I had already found out where the Fed Ex office was, just in case.

Chapter Twelve

Father's Day, June 20th, was also the last day of spring. Summer would start the next day. As I sat by the pool at the Drayson Center on the Loma Linda University Campus, I thought, "Every day so far has been like summer; I guess there won't be any parades or anything today to salute the occasion."

Sitting there in the warm Loma Linda sun, I was remembering those chilly days back in Wisconsin when the groundhog and I both were trying to figure out what to do. Thinking about that self-imposed crash course in prostate cancer, from which I'd graduated back in February, I recalled the exact moment that I turned the corner in my decision making.

The choice was locked in back in February, as I read an email received from a former proton patient, Ed Souder, a World War II hero who'd received the Purple Heart. At age 79, he was diagnosed with prostate cancer. Ed was faced with his biggest battle since he'd huddled with his buddies in that foxhole just inside Germany in 1943. He had been told by doctors there was not much that could be done about his cancer except to give him hormones to slow the growth and drugs to reduce pain, and he was told his time was limited.

Then four years later, at age 83, and after being treated at Loma Linda, he was still going strong - and sent me this email:

"Bill: Without doubt - the one and only place in the USA to go for eradication of Prostate Cancer is Loma Linda, Ca. I was diagnosed in July 2000 with a PSA of 29.7, then put on Lupron and they were all set to do the seed stuff when I learned about Loma Linda from a former student I taught back in 1956 in Kalispell, Mt. He came to visit me in Minneapolis and after a three hour lunch, I did some further checking, I decided that LLUMC was for me.

"I didn't know anyone at LLUMC so wrote an email letter to a Dr. Rossi and two days later got a return message saying that if I had enough insurance and would wait until his schedule opened up some—he would be happy to be my doctor. His name was Dr. Carl Rossi. I had a Gleason rating of 6 and since it was said that I had cancer which had escaped the capsule - I would be treated with 16 proton treatments and then 28 photon treatments to hit the areas under and around the prostate.

You will hear about the care each person gets while there - and it is truly a miracle. In a very personal and kindly way you are a member of their family and that close association makes your treatment a thing of pure joy. They make the athletic facility there available to each radiation patient and it is truly a state-of- the-art place. I hope you will call me by phone next week and we can talk further about why Loma Linda is the ONLY place I would suggest for a fellow from Wisconsin.

"I look forward to further word from you and so let me be your personal guide in this bad time in your life.

Please contact me soon–
Sincerely, Ed Souder"

Later, I learned Ed had become known as "The Orchid Man." He handed out orchids at his last support group meeting, and would occasionally send orchids to Nurse Sharon Hoyle, whom he and others, refer to as "Florence Nightingale."

Father's Day was a success for me, spending it alone, but not *really* alone. Somehow I felt Ed was there with me, smiling in the knowledge that his email had such impact. I also felt

Tori Lou's presence knowing that, at least for a moment back home, she'd thought of me on this special day.

By Monday, June 21st, this had become my routine: Get up, check e-mail, work on web designs, put on shorts, t-shirt and sandals. Then, walk to the hospital; go in my "special" entrance by the emergency room and down the elevator one floor to Level "B."

I would chat with other patients, read last month's Newsweek magazine, wait for my name to be called, and then go into the little changing room. Wrestling with the hospital gown, I would eventually get it tied behind my neck, then march into Gantry Three.

Chapter Thirteen

On June 29th, I took a road trip to Bel Air to visit a friend I had met, of all places, on the Internet and whom I had known for several years. While we'd become long distance friends via our computers, we had no idea if or when we'd ever actually meet.

"You'll have to tell the guard at the gate who you are and he will let you in," Tobyann told me over my cell phone.

"Okay," I answered, "And, I really have to go to the bathroom. There aren't any gas stations around here," I told her, as I completed my hour-and-a-half drive from Loma Linda to this exclusive, gated community nestled in the hills between Hollywood and Santa Monica, just a mile from the famed Getty Museum.

"Well, we have bathrooms," she laughed, "see you in a few minutes."

I got there just moments after their housekeeper had arrived and she had taken the only obvious parking spot right in front of the house, so I parked in front of the neighboring house.

"That's okay," Tobyann explained, "They are hardly ever there. It's the Hungarian Consulate. Oh, there's a bathroom right down that hall."

An art connoisseur and former professional ballroom dancer, Tobyann teaches dance, is an art collector, decorator, semi-professional shopper and an admitted chocoholic. Her husband Lester, conservatively convivial, is a partner in a large CPA firm in West Los Angeles.

He has a curriculum vitae longer than the credits at the end of a Harry Potter movie. He's an expert in forensic accounting and financial management. Among his firm's clients are many actors, producers, directors, and writers.

I visited Lester's office and spent almost two hours with him and one of his partners analyzing their web site and making some suggestions. They actually took notes. I met David, a long-time employee of the firm, who is one of the men I talked with, back in February, as I tried to make a decision about which type of cancer treatment was best for me. He had survived prostate cancer a few years before, having successfully undergone surgery. I also met their office manager, who was the personal assistant to George Burns, until George died at age 100.

That evening we had dinner and I drove back to Loma Linda. Despite getting on the wrong freeway and ending up in Pasadena, a bit out of the way, I still made it back in less time than it had taken to get to Bel Air that morning, because the best time to travel in Southern California is late at night, when the traffic is not quite as heavy.

So, how did I come to meet these folks from Bel Air over the Internet? We haven't really been able to figure it out.

About four years earlier, on a Saturday morning, in an attempt by one of us to send an instant message, all of a sudden we appeared on each others' computers.

"Are you the person in Nashville I was chatting with the other day?" I asked.

"No, are you one of my husband's clients?" the woman guessed.

"I don't think so," I said, sounding pretty sure of that.

"Where are you? And . . . *who* are you?" came the response.

We joked about how weird the Internet can be sometimes and exchanged a few lol's (Internet shorthand for "laughing out loud"). I learned this mystery person, Tobyann, and her husband Lester, lived in California. She had heard of Wisconsin, but had never been there. After that we chatted fairly often.

Once in awhile Tori Lou would talk with her on line. Tobyann had a friend who ran a Beanie Baby store where she could get a good deal, and one year around Christmas she sent a huge box of Beanie Babies to Tori Lou.

For whatever reason, she had sent them by first class mail and spent about twenty-seven dollars on postage!

"You're crazy," I emailed her. "Why didn't you send the package UPS? And, the way you taped it up, you must have spent ten bucks on tape!"

"I wanted to make sure it got there on time and in one piece," she explained, apparently forgetting that Beanies are pretty much unbreakable.

Chapter Fourteen

All of a sudden, it was the end of June! And, on that 30th day of the Month of Gloom, I had something to celebrate. I had completed treatment number 22 with 22 more to go. I was at the halfway mark!

While I was not officially on the Atkins Diet, I had been "watching my carbs." But, this was a special occasion! At Gerrard's Market in Redlands, my new favorite market, which featured the best meat and seafood department I'd ever seen, I spotted a small loaf of freshly baked French bread.

"Yes, that's how I will celebrate." I decided to treat myself to a couple of slices of fresh French bread, along with a nice New York strip steak I picked out with help from the butcher. This would indeed be a special night!

After hurrying back to San Lucas Drive with my culinary treasures, I fired up the stove. Really hot pan, a little salt, four minutes on each side. Wow, what a steak!

The baby portabella mushrooms sautéed in sherry and a few small ripe cherry tomatoes rounded out this perfect meal of celebration.

I had so looked forward to the French bread, I saved it for last. Kind of a crusty dessert.

I placed the smallish, but beautiful loaf on the cutting board, and with one smooth stroke that Julia Childs would have applauded, I sliced a perfect eighth-inch slice . . . off the end of my thumb!

My first thought was, "Oh, no Lorraine's gonna kill me. I'm getting blood all over her duplex." My second thought was, "Now what do I do?"

With my hand held high over my head and a wad of gauze and paper towel wrapped around it, I walked to the emergency room using the same route I had taken earlier in the day when going for my twenty-second treatment. It was about six-thirty in the evening and the emergency room was packed.

Just before entering the building, I saw a helicopter coming in for a landing on the roof. Loma Linda is one of the top trauma centers in Southern California and the patients who come in by copter get treated right away. But, the seventh floor trauma center operates at a different level than the "cut thumb" department down on the first floor.

They were very busy, and since my bleeding had stopped and I wasn't in any immediate danger, I had to wait my turn.

I talked for awhile with a guy who appeared to be about twenty and had fallen off his bicycle. He was scuffed up and had hurt his shoulder. I tried to console him by telling him horror stories of how Tori Lou flipped her bike one time and had to have stitches. It didn't seem to help much; he continued to grimace as he was called into the exam room just ahead of me.

It was almost two hours before either the bike rider or I finally got to see someone for treatment. A student nurse applied my first bandage around eight-thirty P.M. and it was almost eleven by the time I'd had my dressing changed twice, got a tetanus shot, and was ready to go.

While I couldn't wait to go home and kick that loaf of bread across the room, I first had to take prescriptions up to the hospital's 24-hour pharmacy and wait for them. The antibiotics were a must, and the pain pills might come in handy later. It was in the waiting area of the pharmacy when I had another of those *I must be here for a reason* moments.

Handing the pharmacist my prescriptions, I was told it would be about ten minutes. I sat down and tried to stay awake, and as my head started to nod, a man and woman came in with a prescription to be filled.

"This is for my son," the woman said to the pharmacist, "He's downstairs. He fell off his bike."

"How's he doing?" I asked the dad, "I came in at the same time." I held up my thumb to show him why I was there. The dad squinted in sympathy at the sight of my big white bandage.

"He's okay. He bruised his shoulder pretty bad, but it wasn't dislocated," he said. "How'd you do that?" the man asked.

"I cut it slicing bread," I frowned, "I was celebrating the halfway mark of my proton radiation treatment for prostate cancer here at Loma Linda." I told him a little about the procedure.

Just like the New Yorker who's never been to the Statue of Liberty, this man knew very little about proton radiation, at that time available at only three places in the U.S., including the very building we were in.

He appeared to be in his mid-fifties and explained that his father had died of prostate cancer. He had not had a PSA test for a couple of years. By the time the pharmacist had my prescription ready, I'd convinced him that he must get a new PSA test soon and learn more about proton treatment.

"Maybe I cut my thumb for a reason," I said, at the risk of sounding too dramatic.

"You may be right," he said. "Thank you very much."

"Maybe your son crashed his bike for a reason," I added, forgetting that it doesn't necessarily take *two* bad things to make one good thing happen.

The man closed his eyes, shook his head slowly, and let out a deep breath. As a Dad, I understood that to mean, "My kid did a dumb thing, but I still love him, and maybe it *did* happen for a reason."

I went home and tried a homemaker's tip I'd heard a long time ago to clean up the blood I'd gotten on Lorraine's carpet. I used shampoo and it took the blood right out! My anger at the loaf of bread had subsided, so I refrained from kicking it. But, I did give it a pretty hard toss into the plastic-lined waste basket. For the rest of my life, every time I use a serrated knife, I will remember that 22nd proton treatment.

I'd seen a sign at the Drayson Center pool that said you can't go in with any bandages. As I fell asleep that night, with the help of a pain pill, I hoped to have the bandage off by the time Tori Lou arrived so we could go swimming together.

Chapter Fifteen

On the night of the Fourth of July, I watched the New York City fireworks on TV and listened to the San Bernardino fireworks. They were going off across the way behind the duplex.

I could not see the bursts from the deck, but I could hear them, and see some of the flashes from the larger explosions, reflecting off the windows of the Medical Center building across the way.

The next day, July 5th, I talked to Tori Lou. It was the day before her flight to California.

"How were the big fireworks in Madison?" I asked.

Every year there's an event called Rhythm and Booms. One of the local radio stations plays music that is roughly matched up to the bombs bursting in sky. Folks sit on blankets with boom boxes and mosquito repellant and enjoy the show. It's quite a big deal.

"It got rained out. They're having it tonight." Tori Lou replied.

"Are you going?" I asked.

"I don't think so. I have to finish packing and see some of my friends before I leave," she said.

"Try to get some sleep," I advised, "Remember when you get here, and it's ten o'clock tomorrow night, it will be midnight in Madison."

"So?" she said.

"Good point," I concluded. "I'll pick you up at the Ontario airport at around noon tomorrow. I love you."

"Luvutu," she said, combining the phrase into one fast word.

Chapter Sixteen

Parking Lot Full the sign said, but cars were pulling into the lot across from the America West terminal. "How does this work?" I asked the parking attendant, a guy about eighty-five.

"People are leaving all the time, just come in and drive around until . . . hey, there's one right here on the end." he interrupted himself.

Sure enough a car was backing out not twenty feet from me. I pulled in parked and walked into the terminal. The flight had already arrived, according to the monitor screens lined up in the middle of the baggage pickup area, but no signs of any passengers yet.

I went into the men's room and moments later, as I came out and started to walk toward the baggage area, I heard "Hey, Dad! Over here!"

There she was, skateboard in hand, ready to take Southern California by storm. After a long hug, and a short wait for baggage, we headed west on the "Ten" toward Loma Linda. It was only about a twenty-five minute drive.

"It's a little noisy here on the freeway with the top down," I said.

"What?" said Tori Lou.

"It's a little noisy here on the freeway with the top down!" I repeated. "Careful your cap doesn't blow off!" She had a huge collection of baseball caps, which she'd be adding to in the near future I was sure.

"Oh, yeah!" she said loudly. "Where are the mountains?"

"They're kind of over there," I said pointing to the east apologetically, "June Gloom has been extended into July, so it's a little hazy; but as we get closer to the mountains, they will be easier to see."

"When we get closer to the mountains, they will be easier to see," she restated slowly in a deliberate tone, mimicking my overstatement of the obvious.

"Yeah, you'll see.," I assured her.

"Okay, Dad," she raised one eyebrow, and continued to look around in controlled amazement, quietly fascinated by the passing scene.

Though she was weary from the long flight and lack of sleep the night before, I could tell she was excited to be there and anxious to get to Loma Linda.

"I can't wait to see that tree you sent me a picture of," she said, "the one I said I was going to climb." Tori Lou always preferred participating over watching.

"Can we eat at the place that has the best hamburgers in the world?" she asked.

"We'll see," came the standard Dad answer. "It's called Farmer Boys and it's in Yucaipa."

"Hey, that's where you said there's a skate park," she remembered. "Can I skate if we go there?"

"Not so fast," I smiled. "You can't do everything the first day. And, there's this thing called unpacking."

"Oh, yeah. Do I have a big closet?" her thoughts turning to more domestic concerns.

"You have a huge closet, a big bed and your own bath," I explained, "I think you're really going to like the place."

"Yeah, me too," she replied. "Are we almost there?"

Minutes later the freeway sign came into view, "Loma Linda University Next Exit."

Making the exit onto Anderson Street was more than just a routine escape from the perils of the freeway. Later we would come to realize and appreciate the significance of the turn we were making. It marked the start of a five week sun-drenched sabbatical, during which a dad and his daughter, fifty years his junior, would discover just how much they had in common.

Dad would witness how a teenager could skate fearlessly into unknown territory and make friends just by being herself; gregarious, frighteningly perceptive and sometimes a little fanciful.

She would see how a dad could maintain a positive attitude in the face of adversity; be serious and whimsical at the same time and, sometimes, show an amazing ability to figure things out.

Both would marvel at the geographical generosity of our country; make new friends, young and old, and learn new skills. We pulled into the alley that led to the carport behind the duplex and parked next to Robert's Ford Excursion.

"When can I meet Sebastian?" Tori Lou asked.

"Let's unpack the car first," I urged as I popped open the trunk.

"Yeah, I want to change into something cooler. These sweatpants I wore from Wisconsin are too hot," she said grabbing one of the suitcases. "And, I've got to call Mom and tell her we made it," she added, obviously excited.

We carried the first couple of bags inside and immediately Tori Lou headed for her room to check it out.

"This bed is really soft!" she said as she plopped down atop the big comforter.

"So how do you like the place?" I asked.

"It's like awesome," she said in her best Valley Girl impersonation.

After we settled in a bit, Tori Lou realized she hadn't eaten since a snack in the Phoenix airport during a layover.

"Can we go get the world's greatest hamburger?" she said.

"Sure. Hey, I found out there's a Farmer Boys closer, just up the way on Redlands Avenue," I announced.

"Cool, let's go there," she said putting on one of the baseball caps from her collection.

On the way out to the car she asked, "Is this where you saw the gecko you told me about?" her memory obviously intact, despite the lack of food. "If I see one, can I try to catch it?"

"Well, if you grab one by the tail, the tail comes off." I cautioned "but, then they grow a new one."

She pondered that for a moment and said, "Then I'll have to figure out a better way to grab them."

Days later she finally saw a small gecko, but it was too fast for her to experiment in methods of capture.

On the way to Redlands we turned on the CD player and sang along with Michael Buble's version of "Come Fly With Me." Before we would finally arrive back home in Wisconsin some five weeks and three thousand miles later we would know all the lyrics to that and several other songs, which most teenagers have never heard of, nor learned.

"This cheeseburger's okay, but I don't know if it's the world's greatest," she proclaimed, "but the French fries are great."

Conclusively she added, "But then, they never said they had the world's greatest *cheeseburgers*." Farmer's Boy was off the hook.

When we returned to our home away from home, and pulled into the carport, guess who was in the alley? Neighbor Noreen and the convivial canine Tori Lou had been anxious to meet!

"Sebastian, buddy!" she ran over to the one hundred and sixty pound charmer and wrapped her arms around him. He gave her a slobbery kiss on the elbow and they became instant friends. It was getting late, so she promised Sebastian she'd take him for a walk the next day.

That night Tori Lou slept like a log in her new, soft bed while I drifted off thinking how lucky I was to have her with me and to be just nineteen proton treatments away from completing my therapy. The first twenty-five sessions had gone by quickly and without a hitch.

Chapter Seventeen

July 7th, Tori Lou and I settled into a morning routine. Six-thirty A.M., eight-thirty Central, I got up and made coffee then worked some on my computer. After taking a shower, I put on my usual outfit; t-shirt, shorts and sandals, and walked the four minutes to get my treatment at eight-thirty.

Returning around nine o'clock, I fixed Tori Lou her favorite breakfast of a bagel with peanut butter and we more or less planned our day. I hadn't really thought about what we'd do that first day, but Tori Lou already had an agenda in mind.

"Dad, you know I didn't buy new skateboard shoes before I left, because it would be one more thing to pack," she said analytically, while clicking through the TV channels to find a suitable cartoon, "I figured we could do that when I got here. Can we do that? And, can I go skating at Yucaipa?"

"Don't forget Sebastian . . ." I started to remind her of the walk she had promised him.

"It's pretty hot already; I'll take him for a walk tonight when it's cooler; he'll like that," she said. "Do you know where we can go to look for shoes?"

Having done a little advance research, knowing this shoe search thing would probably come up sooner than later, I told her I knew of a skate shop in Redlands called 'Icon.' They have stores all over the area and it turned out she'd heard of them.

"Awesome, I hope they have my size," she added hopefully.

She'd left her skateboard in the trunk of the car for a quick getaway, whenever the first skating opportunity came up. Skating had become somewhat of an obsession over the past few months and she hadn't skated for over three days!

Although I knew there were probably no colleges offering scholarships in skateboarding, I never tried to discourage her from skating because she loved it so much.

After stopping at 'Icon' and finding the "perfect" pair of Adios shoes, we drove to Yucaipa where we located the park. There were only three kids skating at the time, but as is her nature, Tori Lou struck up some instant friendships. Before we left the skateboard park, she had exchanged cell phone numbers with two boys about her age. Tyler, the skinny talkative one and Wesley, the young comedian.

After skating for about two hours and showing them a couple of skateboard moves they'd never seen a girl do before, we headed out. After a quick stop at the Farmer's Boy drive-thru for a large Coke, we headed to Loma Linda.

At age thirteen, "hanging" with friends is of utmost importance. It doesn't always matter where you are or what you're doing, as long as you're with your buddies; that's what counts. As a Dad, I knew that when kids are with their friends, Dad becomes more or less invisible.

Recognized as the one who drives the car and carries the credit card, Dad's importance is not minimized; it is just modified as the situation dictates. I accepted this role happily, because I remembered vividly when I was a kid and was the same way.

When I was thirteen, "Can Steve go with?" was a common expression my mother and step dad would hear whenever they proposed any sort of outing. One of my closest friends to this day is my buddy Steve Borota, whom I first met in sixth grade. He has lived in Mississippi for years and we have stayed in touch.

Steve is a stockbroker and has managed my mutual fund investments for many years, even though he lives several states away, and the company he works for has an office just a few blocks from my home. Friendships made during the early teen years often prove to be the most lasting.

I doubted that either of Tori Lou's friends, Tyler or Wesley, would be handling her finances fifty years hence; but they would probably stay in touch, at least for awhile.

"I'm going to walk Sebastian; want to come with?" Tori Lou asked me, obviously not at all tired from a couple hours of skating on the Yucaipa's concrete ramps and half pipe (a U-shaped skating area that looks like a huge concrete drainage pipe sliced in half).

"Sure," I said, not quite ready to turn her loose on her own in the relatively unfamiliar neighborhood. "Let's go."

As we opened the gate and started up the

walkway into Sebastian's backyard, he spotted us and ran over to the bench where his leash was kept. He picked it up in his big, slobbery mouth and loped toward Tori Lou. He hadn't forgotten their date.

"Hi, Buddy, ready for your walk?" she asked. With a wag of his huge tail and a little pretend tug-of-war with the leash, he appeared ready.

Because they are bred to rescue mountain climbers in the Alps during blizzards, the hot California climate didn't seem like the perfect habitat for a St. Bernard. But, Sebastian had obviously adapted. He found that the heat was not a problem if he did not walk at a speed of more than one mile per hour. There was slack in his leash throughout the entire walk.

Returning to his yard, Sebastian headed straight for the six-foot diameter inflatable pool which he used primarily as a drinking bowl and he splashed down right in the middle of it. This guy knew how to cool off after a long, slow walk.

One of my favorite pictures of the entire journey turned out to be one of Tori Lou and Sebastian, walking up a sloping street in Loma Linda with a wooden fence to one side, palm trees on the other and mountains in the background.

With both of their backs to the camera, and leash drooping between them, the scene recalled to me the Roy Rogers and Dale Evans song, "Happy trails to you, until we meet again . . ."

It also made me think again of that picture hanging on my office wall back in Wisconsin.

"Don't Fear the Big Dogs–Billy Vancil, Age 9."

That became my watchword when dealing with some of the hierarchy of the business world and now it seemed an appropriate motto as I faced my current challenge. I recalled the first time I used that philosophy in a business situation. The result, for better or worse, determined my career path for the following forty years.

During my first year in college, at Illinois Wesleyan University, I was an art major. I wanted to become a "commercial artist." But, I had done a little radio work in high school, at the local Kewanee, Illinois radio station, WKEI.

So, when time came to look for a summer job back in my home town, following completion of my first year of college, I made applications to a number of places.

I received two offers; one was from the radio station and the other from Brown Sign Company. Sign painter or radio announcer? I had a decision to make. I accepted the position with the sign company.

My first day on the job, I was told to paint a sign for a Laundromat. The sign was to say, "No Dyeing." I finished the sign by the end of the day and took it to the owner of the company, Mr. Brown. By then, I had gotten up the nerve to ask an important question.

"By the way, Mr. Brown," I asked, "How much do I get paid?"

"Oh, you don't get paid," he answered, "You're an apprentice."

I looked Mr. Brown straight in the eye, and said, "No, I'm not . . . I'm a radio announcer."

I accepted the job at WKEI the next day, at a wage of one dollar per hour.

That was my first experience facing up to a "big dog." I stayed in the radio business for over forty years, growing from a dollar-an-hour announcer to Vice-President and General Manager, as well as part-owner, of five radio stations.

Years later, tiring of the corporate rat race, I coincidentally discovered that I could make a "No Dyeing" sign, in seconds, using a computer.

That's when I made a career change and became a graphic artist. I cashed in my part-ownership and management position with the radio stations and started my own company, *Vancil Creative.* Broadcasting went from profession to avocation.

I continue to do some radio-related work, such as commercials, voiceovers and a bit of consulting; but I enjoy the creative design work, and I especially enjoy "being my own boss." If I have a client who bares his teeth, I can walk away, without fear.

Chapter Eighteen

It was July 8th, and the June Gloom had started to dissipate somewhat. Skateboard wheels still spinning from the day before, Tori Lou and I decided to spend the day at the beach. Just an hour from Loma Linda, Seal Beach seemed like it would make a good day-trip. We left right after my morning treatment and were lucky to find a parking place just a half block from the beach.

We walked out to the end of the long pier from which we had a great look back at the expansive sand beach, as well as a nice view of Long Beach to the North and Huntington Beach to the South. Tori Lou could wait no longer to get into the surf.

We found a place to rent a boogie board, which is shorter than a surfboard, and great fun. It was windy at Seal Beach that day and the breeze off the ocean was cool. It's easy to see why Johnny Mountain could generalize about the temps being "cooler at the beach" and "warmer inland."

Of course, it didn't faze the conquering hero- ine from Wisconsin. She tamed the waves as easily as she made friends with Sebastian. We took a break for lunch, and then she did some more boogie boarding. "Next I'm going to learn to surf!" Tori Lou proclaimed.

Almost admitting to being a little tired, she finally agreed to head back home. And then we learned a valuable lesson. It is not wise to try to drive through Orange County at five o'clock in the afternoon.

While it took just one hour to get to the beach, it took three hours to get back. In subsequent trips to places which were more than an hour away, we waited until after dark to head home.

When we got back to our duplex, there was a message from Jerry McAdow, my attorney back in Madison, who had been tracking all the communications with the insurance company.

Despite the two hour time difference, I was confident that I could return the call without fear of waking Jerry. I knew that he always worked late into the evening.

What I found out helped settle my nerves, just a little rattled from the three hour marathon on the freeways. Jerry reported that everything seemed to be going well with the insurance company.

He felt fairly certain they would end up paying for most of my proton radiation treatment, unless something unexpected arose.

We decided to employ "watchful waiting" rather than raise any discussion unnecessarily with the insurance company. "Watchful waiting" is a phrase we learned while doing our investigation of cancer treatments.

It is generally recommended only for men who are quite old, whose cancer is less aggressive; and who are likely to die of something else before the cancer reaches the critical stage. Treatment must be individualized; and "watchful waiting" was not an option I considered, even for a moment.

In addition to the message from Jerry, I received an email from the manager of the home security company in Madison with whom I'd talked over a month ago. He still wanted me to record the phone answering dialog for his company's new system, and had included 15 pages of scripts. Things like, "If you know the extension of the party you're calling enter it now . . ."

I called Inland Empire Recording Studio in Redlands and reserved studio time for the following week.

The next morning we went across the alley to visit Sebastian. Tori Lou would not have time to take him for a walk, as we were going to leave shortly for a daytrip to Palm Springs. Oh, yes, I did have my proton treatment that morning.

Sometimes, it was easy to forget the main purpose of this trip, because the treatments were painless and had become routine.

As we walked into the yard, Sebastian picked up his leash expecting to go for a walk. Tori Lou explained to him that he would have to wait. We spent a few minutes chatting with Noreen and solved one of the big mysteries of life. We not only learned about kumquats; we actually saw and tasted some!

In her yard, Noreen had not only Concord grape vines and lemon trees, but a kumquat tree! Kumquat is one of those things like aardvark and Timbuktu. You hear about it from time to time, but don't know what it is. A kumquat is a small, edible orange-like fruit with an acid pulp and a thin, edible rind. It is the smallest of the citrus fruits. That's what the dictionary says, and that's what we tasted. Not bad.

Noreen said, "If you eat too many, they are bad for your teeth." Her husband is a dentist.

"See you later, Buddy!" Tori Lou shouted to Sebastian as he dropped his leash and sniffed what was left of one of the kumquats.

We took off for the famous getaway place of the movie stars, Palm Springs, just an hour from Loma Linda.

To get there we drove through a mountain pass that was the windiest place I'd ever been.

Hundreds of huge windmills stand like objects from outer space in the valley and on the mountainsides. They harness the constantly strong winds to generate electrical power for the region.

While we didn't see any movie stars, we did see a very cool skateboard park. Very cool and very hot! It was almost 100 degrees and even Tori Lou admitted it was too hot to skate. We had lunch at a restaurant where we could sit outside under "misters" which sprayed a cooling mist into the air, making dining outdoors bearable.

Conveniently located between Loma Linda and Palm Springs is a huge outlet mall, where we stopped on the way back to Loma Linda. Tori Lou got some tank tops and a pair of sandals. She helped me choose a new pair of walking shoes for myself. I started to wonder how many pair of shoes we might be sending home by Fedex when the time came to pack up.

We made one more stop and one more purchase before we got home. We visited a shop in Redlands called Banned, which sells gear for skateboarding, snowboarding *and* surfing. Location, location, location.

My credit card suffered just a minor bruise in that store, as the only thing which Tori Lou saw that was a necessity was another hat for the collection. This one was all white with a stylized "H" on the front (the logo of Hurley, a sporty clothing brand that is popular among skateboarders and surfers.)

This would become Tori Lou's favorite hat and it appears in many of the photos taken during our journey.

Chapter Nineteen

It was July 10th, and I had signed us up for the Saturday morning tour of the Proton Treatment Center. Tori Lou was looking forward to seeing this mysterious place, where Dad went every weekday morning at 8:30.

For almost two hours we toured the facility, including a stop in one of the three treatment rooms in which gantries are used to deliver the proton beam to prostate cancer patients.

The tour guide explained, "The 90-ton, three-story gantries can be rotated 360 degrees to deliver the beam at the precise angle prescribed by the physician. Most of the gantry is concealed by the walls and floor of the treatment room. The patient, lying in his pod, only sees the front of the proton nozzle rotating prior to treatment."

Then he opened a pair of doors and revealed the huge gyroscope looking assemblage of working parts called the gantry. This behemoth was something you'd expect to see inside the lower deck of an aircraft carrier or something. All those times I'd climbed into my pod, I never realized what a huge piece of technology was quietly at work behind the walls of the treatment room.

The guide further explained, "Each treatment takes from 20 to 40 minutes. Most of the time is spent aligning the patient to ensure that the proton beam is delivered to the precise location prescribed in the treatment plan. Actual proton beam delivery takes approximately one minute, during which time the patient feels nothing."

Tori Lou had seen the two things she was most curious about; the pod and the gantry. I had heard most of this before, so we worked our way to the back of the group. She was anxious to move on to other things. As we quietly exited through the passageway I'd grown so familiar with, we heard the guide continuing, "Physicians at the Loma Linda proton facility can deliver radiation precisely to an irregular three-dimensional volume in any anatomic location within a patient. This provides physicians with a better method for delivering radiation therapy."

We decided it was time to check out another skate park. One of the closer ones was the park at Upland. Built in 2002, it brought a long-awaited skate park back to Upland after the legendary, original Upland Pipeline closed in 1988. The new park has a 22 foot full pipe, a 12 foot bowl and a great street course.

There were some pretty good skaters there and we watched for awhile, but it was really crowded and hot that day, so we decided to make a run down to Orange and visit the Vans indoor park at the "The Block," a big mall in Orange.

Vans Skatepark is one of the biggest and most popular in Southern California. Aside from the fact that helmet, knee pads and elbow pads are required, Tori Lou thought it was the coolest place she'd ever seen. Operated by the huge shoe manufacturer Vans, it had become sacred ground for serious Orange County skateboarders in recent years. It featured an 80-foot vertical ramp and a 20,000 square foot pro street course.

The Combi Pool at Vans is a replica of the original Upland Pipeline skate park of the '80s and known as one of the best pools in skateboarding history. This is where Tori Lou started skating with the "big dogs." And, at least in this Dad's totally unbiased opinion, she was becoming a terrific skater.

It was not uncommon to hear a spectator, watching from the mezzanine overlooking the street course to say, "Wow, that's a girl?"

Some of the skaters, several of them also girls, were closer to professional caliber skaters than any we'd seen so far. We found out during our four or five subsequent visits to Vans, that some actually were professionals.

Tori Lou made friends right away with some younger kids and gave them some pointers on skating. She also got to know Martin Aparijo, who was one of the worlds' top ranked inline skaters and BMX bikers in the late 80s. Martin teaches skateboarding at Vans, but when he saw Tori Lou skate he said, "You don't really need lessons, you've got the natural moves. You just need to skate and practice and hang out with good skaters. I'll skate with you anytime; I'm here most all the time."

I did not relate his later comment to Tori Lou, for fear her head would swell too much to fit in the required helmet. Martin told me during a break, "If she could skate all the time in parks like this, with practice, I think she could be a world-class skater within a few years."

I wondered, "How many pairs of skate shoes would it take, placed end-to-end, to reach from here to World-Class?"

Tori Lou signed up for a Vans membership, so she'd get a discount every time she came back, which she was sure would be often.
As I watched her skate in this higher level environment, I could see her confidence and skill level increasing noticeably.

We took a break to have lunch at Johnny Rocket's, a '50s throwback diner in the mall. They had a replica jukebox in each booth and Tori Lou flipped through the selections testing Dad's knowledge of oldies.

"Who did *Book of Love?*" she asked.

"Monotones," I answered.

"*There Goes My Baby?*" she asked.

"Drifters," I replied.

"*Runaway?*"

"Del Shannon."

"Hey, here's our food," she said, putting the quiz on hold. "Don't tell the guys at Farmer Boys, but this might be the best burger in the world," she said as she bit into the juicy one-third pounder.

"Mroo dud *Craliformnia Jreemen?*" she asked.

"Mommas and Poppas," I laughed, "Don't talk with your mouth full.

"Shorry," she drooled.

Chapter Twenty

Monday, July 12th, was my day to visit the studio in Redlands to record the telephone answering scripts. A quiet young man named Sean was my engineer for the session. Sean set up the microphone, I put on the headphones, and he started the digital recording device.

"You have reached the voice mail system of . . ."

"Thank you for your patience. If you would like to leave a message . . ."

"If you are calling to report an emergency . . ."

"Due to inclement weather, our office is temporarily closed . . ."

"To hear these options again, please press pound . . ."

On it went all fifteen pages worth. Finally, I was finished reading and Sean set up the equipment to transfer the messages onto a CD, which I would send overnight to the client.

To do this, we had to sit patiently, and listen to all the messages, one at a time, as they were "burned" onto the CD in "real time." No speeding up this process.

Sean didn't talk much, but right near the end of the session, the soft-spoken born-and-raised Californian asked me, "What's *inclement* weather?"

I chuckled, knowing he was serious.

"It's when the weather is so bad you can't go to work," I explained.

"Hmm, I've never heard that word before," he said, raising his eyebrows.

"I don't think Johnny Mountain ever heard it before either," I said, "It's a Wisconsin thing."

The next day we were back at The Block in Orange, featuring Vans Skatepark, Johnny Rocket's, and lots of cool stores. This was clearly Tori Lou's kind of place. She was holding her own. Skating with the "big dogs," making friends, and of course, buying more shoes.

"I totally must have those checkered slip-ons," she proclaimed as we walked through the Vans skate store on the way to the skating area.

"You're already into next week's allowance," I reminded her.

"Can we push it ahead another week? Those are really cool shoes. I've seen them on the Vans web site," she pleaded.

"I suppose," I gave in, feigning exasperation. They were pretty cool shoes. I even tried on a pair myself, but they did not have the narrow width I require. Thank goodness I'm hard to fit, or I'd have two shoe addicts on my hands.

One of her many pairs of shoes, specifically the sandals she picked up at the mall near Palm Springs, played an unexpected role in some matchmaking one afternoon.

We were just hanging out at home. I was catching up on some work on the computer and Tori Lou was sitting out on the deck, talking long distance by cell phone with a friend back in Wisconsin. It was the usual conversation, of which Dad only hears one side.

"Hey . . . Whazzup . . . Nothin' . . . Yeah . . . Cool . . ."

I was concentrating on my work and not paying much attention, so I didn't hear her go out the door. I was surprised when about ten minutes later the door opened and she walked in and made her announcement, "I have a couple of new friends. They're coming over later."

"So, who are these friends, and how did you meet them?" I asked.

"Chris is 13, same as me, and his brother Devon is 10. They're really cool and I met them because my sandal fell off," she explained.

"How's that?" I asked. "Run that by me again."

"Well, I was sitting on the deck talking on the phone to Taz back home," she said, "and I was dangling my foot over the edge and my sandal fell off. So, I had to go down to get it."

"And . . ." I urged her to go on.

She explained that Chris was skating past on his inline skates, just as she happened to be saying something to Taz about inline skating.

Seizing the moment, Chris stopped and said, "Did I hear you say something about inline?"

Not a bad opening line. Better than, "Don't your sandals fit right?"

I couldn't help but recall how I'd met a friend in similar fashion during a trip to Europe with my mother and stepfather. Our bus tour had included a three day stopover in Rome.

While I remember seeing the Coliseum, the Spanish Stairs, Sistine Chapel, St. Peter's Basilica and other famous landmarks; what I remember most is meeting a friend about my age.

We were staying in a hotel in the center of the city. Our room was on the fifth floor. From the window in our room, I could look down into a courtyard just across the narrow street. A kid was playing, bouncing a ball against the courtyard wall. I waved to him; he waved back and smiled.

I decided to try and make friends with him, so I tossed a note out the window. I had folded the paper several times to give it enough weight so it would fall to its intended target, and not blow out into the Tyrrhenian Sea.

The note read, "I'm Bill from the United States, how are you?" or something equally profound. I hadn't considered how he might respond. First, he probably didn't speak English; and second, how could he possibly throw a folded note back up to me on the fifth floor?

Taking a bold, forward approach, I tossed down another note. "May I come down and meet you?" After looking back up at me, the boy ran inside with the message. I found out later, he was calling upon his mom for translation. When he returned to the courtyard, he looked up again. With a big smile and an exaggerated arm signal, he motioned to me to come down.

I took the slow, creaky elevator down to the hotel lobby and made my way out onto the street. I nervously knocked on the courtyard door. The boy and his mom came to greet me. He spoke no English, she spoke a little. We exchanged polite smiles and some fragmented, clumsily translated chit chat. I learned his name was Sandro Berardi and he was two years younger than I. We exchanged addresses and a promise to keep in touch, and then I went back to my hotel.

Sandro and I remained "pen pals" for a couple of years following that brief encounter; then lost touch. I've thought of looking him up, if and when I might return to Rome. I wonder if he would remember me. I wonder if he's having his PSA test done on a regular basis. I hope so.

As I recall that experience, it reinforces my understanding of the craving that teenagers have for being with kids their same age.

And, as a result, I've become more tolerant of Tori Lou when she asks, "Can I bring a friend?"

It was a shame that Tori Lou met Chris and Devon so near the end of our stay in Loma Linda, or they would've had more time together. But the short time they did have was fun.

We took them to Yucaipa skating once and a couple of times to the Drayson Center swimming pool as our guests.

Long after our trip was finished and we'd returned to Madison, Chris still called Tori Lou on her cell phone just to say, "Hi." During one of the calls, he informed Tori Lou that he was taking Sebastian for walks and feeding him while Noreen was on vacation.

It made Tori Lou feel good, because she had introduced Chris and Sebastian. Even though this small friendly kid and large friendly dog lived just a block apart, it took a kid from 2,000 miles away to get them together.

Would this be a friendship that would last?

Time will tell. Some of my early friendships have endured to this day, as the story of our next outing will attest.

Chapter Twenty-One

It had been penciled on the calendar since before Tori Lou arrived in Loma Linda. I had contacted friends in San Diego and finagled an invitation to visit them on the weekend of July 17–18. We'd been friends for over forty years; having worked together in radio in the '60s. While we had stayed in touch over the years, we had not seen each other in over twenty years. I remembered back . . .

"It's six-twenty-five, on a cloudy Saturday morning, time to get up and get going with Bobby Vee and his big hit, *Devil or Angel* right here on W-P-E-O . . . The Pulse of Peoria!" I gushed out, in my phony 19-going-on-35 radio voice.

This was my summer job in Peoria, Illinois in 1960. Radio announcing was something I had gotten into sort of by accident; but it was the stepping stone into a broadcast management career that lasted 40 years, side-tracking me from what I really should have been doing all those four decades. The Program Director at WPEO, "Rapid Robert" Edwards introduced me to a bright young high school student who was going to be working part time at the station. He was Clark Anthony.

Clark (his real full name is Clark Anthony Burlingame) was only 14, just starting high school, and had obtained a special permit to work after school and weekends. I wasn't sure what he was going to do at WPEO, but he seemed like a nice kid and I showed him around the station, which was on the second floor of a rundown Peoria office building and consisted of two small studios, an office or two and a Dr. Pepper machine.

Not long after Clark started working at WPEO, I transferred to Augustana College in Rock Island, Illinois and got a job at KSTT, the powerhouse Top Forty station of the Quad-Cities. Two years later, I was on the air doing my 21-going-on-37 phony radio delivery:

"It's 10:15 on a sunny Monday morning, time to do the *Loco-Motion* with Little Eva on K-S-T-T, The Quad-Cities' Home of the Good Guys!"

"There's someone here to see you," the voice on the intercom cackled into the studio, as I turned off the microphone.

"I told him you were on the air, but he says you know him. His name is Clark Burlingame."

"You're kidding," I said, "Send him in. That's Clark Anthony! He must have gotten his driver's license. Tell him to come into the studio."

"My parents decided to move here from Peoria," Clark explained. "And, I thought you might need some help."

By then, I'd become Program Director of KSTT and I hired Clark on the spot. Later we'd try to figure out what he would do. In reminiscing forty years later, neither of us could remember exactly what he did do, but I remember he was very good at it. After graduating from Rock Island High School, Clark went to Augustana College and continued to work at KSTT, becoming one of its most popular personalities.

In the late '60s, with Viet Nam at a fever pitch, Clark was drafted into the Marines and, as luck would have it, was assigned to do Armed Forces Radio in Southern California.

When Tori Lou and I arrived at his home in San Diego for our visit, it was easy to see why he and his wife Kaye, whom he'd married back in the Quad-Cities, chose to stay in San Diego once his tour of duty ended.

They gave us a tour of the area, driving out to Point Loma for a marvelous view of the bay and city. Then we drove downtown past PETCO Park where the Padres play; we saw the San Diego Zoo and the aircraft carrier, USS Midway.

For many years, Clark was the mid-day host on one of San Diego's most popular stations, KFMB and also did newscasts on KFMB-TV. As I had done, he had then chosen to start his own business, and for the past several years had been enjoying a career as a free-lance announcer.

His voice has been used on commercials for clients like Olympus, Toyota, San Diego Zoo, Tosco and Sea World. It was his connection with Sea World that enabled him to get a couple of passes for Tori Lou and I to visit there, which we would do on Sunday before heading back to Loma Linda.

We spent an enjoyable Saturday evening with our friends; three adults reminisced and Tori Lou enjoyed the swimming pool. The next morning, after a breakfast that could have served the Padres bullpen staff, we headed off for Sea World, just five minutes from Clark and Kaye's home.

The Sea World passes Clark had gotten for us, were all inclusive, except for food, so we could do anything we wanted. The first attraction we chose was a "4-Dimensional" film called "The Haunted Lighthouse."

As the attendant released the satin rope barrier to allow our group to enter the theatre, we heard a friendly but authoritative voice boom out from speakers somewhere in the ceiling.

"In order to make room for your fellow audience members, please move to the center of the theatre and fill all available seats . . ." the comforting, but commanding instructions continued.

"Hey, Lou! That's Clark," I said.

"Really, where?" she asked, looking around at the seats behind us.

"In the ceiling," I said, "That's his voice telling us where to sit."

"No, way. The Clark we had breakfast with?" she questioned, "no, that's not him."

After hearing Clark guide us, over loudspeakers, through several areas of this aquatic wonderland, Tori Lou was finally convinced that it really was Clark. But, she did get a little upset with his recorded announcement which told us, "Journey to Atlantis is experiencing technical difficulties and is temporarily closing for repairs . . ." We had been standing in line for over an hour to ride this new attraction which Sea World had been promoting heavily.

It was quite a disappointment. After all, this new thrill ride had promised to take us to "uncharted waters where mysterious mists and unpredictable drops lurk around every turn!"

It was going to "twist us around serpentine turns, plunge us down eight stories of adrenaline-pumping exhilaration and drench us in mystery!" Oh, well, maybe next time. Everything else was fabulous at Sea World.

Using our newly-acquired technique of coming home late to avoid traffic jams as an excuse to stay as late as possible, we left just as the nightly fireworks display began. We made it back to Loma Linda in less than two hours.

On the way home, before she dozed off, Tori Lou told me how much she enjoyed meeting Clark and Kaye.

It was always that way with Tori Lou.

Whenever we visited places where I introduced her to friends of mine, she always pointed to them as the highlight of the visit.

Our human San Diego friends should feel honored to rank even higher than Shamu, Sea World's famous black and white killer whale.

Chapter Twenty-Two

The following week was a mixture of walking Sebastian, Tori Lou playing with her new friends, going to Van's to skate again, swimming at the Drayson Center, driving up into the mountains to visit Lake Gregory.

About one hour in time and 4,000 feet away in elevation, Lake Gregory is a small community nestled in the San Bernardino Mountains, with narrow streets featuring souvenir shops, realty offices and art galleries.

And, then there's the lake, man-made and small by Wisconsin standards; but we enjoyed the clean water and cooler air as we paddled around on flotation boards which looked like surfboards without fins. Tori Lou went down the waterslide about twenty times.

"Come on Dad, it's fun!" begged Tori Lou, "just do it once."

I gave in and started climbing the long log stairs that wound up the hillside to the top of the slide. The slide looked longer and faster with each step and I kept asking myself, "Why am I doing this?" I knew why.

At the bottom, Tori Lou was all smiles as I climbed out of the splash down area, "See, that wasn't so bad was it?" she asked.

As I walked toward the lifeguard station to get something to blot the blood from my non-life threatening scrapes to both elbows and one knee, I said, "Now, you know what unconditional love is; but one time down the slide is plenty." It was fun, but I didn't want to risk a more serious scrape. Tori Lou seemed satisfied that again, Dad had succumbed to her unflinching insistence.

On Wednesday, July 21st, I had my follow-up meeting with Dr. Baldwin, the surgeon who had performed the laparoscopic surgery prior to starting the proton therapy.

It did not seem possible that nine weeks had passed since the surgery. Dr. Baldwin said everything looked fine. Right after the surgery he had told me he was going on a vacation to hike from the South Rim to the North Rim of the Grand Canyon, so I asked him how that went.

"It was great. If you visit the canyon on your way home to Wisconsin, make sure to visit the North Rim. It's a much better view than from the South," he urged.

I said we would; but later we decided to go home a different route–up the coast to San Francisco and back on Interstate 80, missing the Grand Canyon.

This was the second time in several months that I had not taken the advice of a surgeon, and chose a different path. Although, in this case, it was not a life-altering decision.

"Hey, dad! I was just watching this show on TV called *Switched* and there was a girl from the Midwest switching places with a girl from California who is a surfer," Lou said excitedly, "When am I going to have my surfing lesson?"

"Come in the office; I saved a link to a website for a place that gives lessons," I answered. "Let's check it out."

I clicked on the web address. "Here it is, *Surf City Surfing Lessons*," I said, "operated by Kim Hamrock, 2002 World Champion Women's Long Board. They give lessons down at Newport."

"Wow!" Tori Lou exclaimed, pointing at the website as I scrolled down the computer screen. "There's the girl I just saw on TV! It's Kim's daughter, Margeaux!"

A little further down the screen, we saw Kim's son, Chris, who was described as an avid "skateboarder and surfer." Turned out he was not only avid, but a pro at both. He's the one who ended up giving Tori Lou her first surfing lesson.

When I talked to Kim later that day on the phone, she suggested that because of Tori Lou's proficiency in skateboarding and snowboarding that she'd be a quick learner with Chris as her mentor.

So we arranged for a lesson that coming Saturday, July 24th. The only hitch was, as Kim explained, "We have to give our lessons early because after nine or nine-thirty A.M. the beach is closed to surfing."

Chapter Twenty-Three

"Wake up, Surfer Girl, it's four-thirty A.M.," I said, poking my head into Tori Lou's bedroom. Then I added, hoping to make it less painful to roll out into the darkness, "six-thirty Central." It didn't make it any easier. She was used to sleeping until after nine when I'd return from my proton treatment.

But, this was Saturday and there was no treatment scheduled. It was, however, her opportunity to hit the surf so she gladly, but slowly, rolled out of bed–earlier than at any time since school had ended for the summer a few weeks before.

We were to meet Chris Hamrock at Life Guard Station #7 on the main drag in Newport Beach, right next to the huge wooden pier. We got there at 6:45 and he pulled in about five minutes later. Chris and Tori Lou wiggled into the wetsuits that Surf City provided and, surfboards balanced atop their heads, walked onto the chilled, sparsely populated beach.

There were about ten surfers in the water, but not many souls on the sand, except for a gathering of seagulls picking up after the previous day's litterbugs.

Later the headcount would change dramatically, as the temps rose and the Saturday crowd shuffled in.

The first hour of the surf lesson was conducted on the beach, with Chris building models of waves and surf in the sand. From a distance, it looked like two kids building a castle, but actually they were building a friendship.

Chris explained how waves form and what to look for as they roll in, how to handle yourself if caught in a riptide, how to swim into the waves, judge them and take them on. He showed her how to grip the board and move to a standing position. He reminded her to pick out a landmark on shore in order to know her location in regard to the beach while in the surf.

After an hour or so, of "Classroom in the Sand" instruction, they headed into the water. It was a little after seven A.M., still somewhat cool with the breeze coming in off the Pacific; and the surf had picked up a bit since we first arrived.

They paddled out about two hundred feet from shore and then started drifting and watching for the right wave upon which Tori Lou would make her first attempt.

"Here comes one!" I heard her yell to Chris.

"Yeah, okay, go easy, you can get it!" he encouraged her.

With a little turn of the board and a quick push-up, feet sliding forward, she was actually standing up!

After a momentary wobble, she rode the board all the way in–with knees bent, arms extended and a smile shining bright enough to burn through the morning haze which lingered over Newport Beach.

As these two were laughing and learning in the surf, I was watching, and enjoying the arrival of sunshine. Then I noticed someone else was watching. He had his jeans rolled up to just below the knee for walking on the beach and was carrying a huge camera, with a lens almost as long as one of Lou's skateboards.

As he walked by, I said, "Hi" and he stopped to talk for a moment. He told me he was John Gertz, a professional photographer from South Beach, Florida and that he had rented an RV in order to travel up and down the West Coast for a few weeks of taking pictures for his portfolio.

"I specialize in people pictures," he said. "I do a lot of fashion shots and work with actors and models mostly." He had rented the RV in Los Angeles and had already visited Oregon, Washington, Idaho and Nevada. He was wrapping up his final week in California and that day he decided to get some shots of folks having fun at the beach, and maybe take a little break from work and enjoy the sunshine himself.

"Check out those two over there," I said, pointing to Chris and Tori Lou. "That kid's mom is a world champion surfer and he's teaching my daughter how to surf. It's her first lesson."

He was apparently impressed, probably not so much that I had fathered one of these potential models; but because one of them was of championship stock, I suspect. Wearing their wet suits and wide smiles, they did look strikingly photogenic.

John took dozens of pictures of them, together and separate, and said he would give us all the pictures on a CD, if we would sign a release to allow him to use the pictures in his portfolio. In the photo business, that's called "pictures for pictures." He said he'd even create the disk on the computer in his RV and we could take it with us. It was an easy deal to agree to.

Chris had signed such releases before, being a much-photographed skateboarder; Tori Lou thought she was on a fast track to becoming a super model. I cautioned her not to get her hopes up, but left the door open by under-stating, "You never know what the future holds."

Chris had to leave, so he packed up his gear and headed back to "Surf City." He promised to get in touch with Tori Lou, so they could do some skateboarding before her stay in south-ern California ended. John Gertz decided to put down his camera and have some fun. "The surf's really good today! Want to rent some boogie boards, Tori Lou?"

After thinking about it for about three or four seconds, she said "Are you kidding? Sure!"

After about two hours of boogie boarding, we had dinner with John at The Crab Cooker. Then he headed off down toward Laguna Beach, hoping he would find a place to park his rented RV. He vowed to keep in touch with us.

We, again wisely, waited until after dark before getting on the freeway. It was a little congested, being a Saturday, but we made it back to Loma Linda in just over an hour, tired but happy.

Chapter Twenty-Four

It was Monday morning, July 26, and the start of our final week in Loma Linda. Time had flown by quickly. It was hard to believe that I had only six treatments remaining.

"Hey Tim," I said as I walked into Gantry 3 for the thirty-ninth time, "do you think I could double-up on treatments one day this week so my last one will be on Friday instead of Monday? It'll give us a jump on the long drive home to Wisconsin."

I was half-hoping that he'd say, "No," so we'd have an extra weekend in Loma Linda; but I was pleased to hear him say, "Sure, why don't you come in at your regular time, 8:30 on Thursday morning, and I'll schedule you for another treatment at 4:30 in the afternoon. You need at least six hours between the sessions."

There was a bit of strategy in my plan to double-up on Thursday. Tori Lou and I had been contemplating the different routes we might take to get back to Madison. The original plan was to return the same way I got there; back through Las Vegas, across the heart of Utah, into the Colorado Rockies, through Vail and Denver.

That would have been the most direct route, but I had an alternate plan–a route which would add several hundred miles to the trip but maybe make it even more interesting.

"If we took a couple extra days to get home," I had told her a week or so before, "we could drive up the coast to San Francisco, spend a whole day there and go back through Reno and Cheyenne.

I had secretly dreamed of driving up the Big Sur coastline, with the top down, triumphantly crossing the Bixby Creek Bridge and ceremoniously pushing the imaginary cancer gremlins over the rail.

Tori Lou offered a qualified agreement to my plan. "As long as we can get home by the day I told my friends we'd be there," she articulated.

As you'd expect of most 13-year-olds, she was becoming anxious to see her friends back home.

We had agreed on Saturday, August 6th, as the day we'd arrive back in Madison. I figured she was more concerned with the estimated date of arrival, which she had promoted to her friends, than how many days we'd spend on the road.

I had calculated that by leaving on Saturday morning, instead of Monday, we could gain the two extra days up front and still get home on schedule. City by the Bay, here we come!

Planning ahead, I had gone onto the internet and made a reservation at the Sea Coast Lodge in San Simeon, just a few miles from the Hearst Castle, which was going to be our first stop on our trek back to Wisconsin.

Monday night, July 26th, we invited Robert and Martha to come up to our place for dinner. They were about to leave for Abilene the next morning, so this was kind of a 'going-away get together.' Robert brought the small gas grill he'd bought a few weeks earlier and set it up out on our deck. Tori Lou and I had not acquired a grill, because our vehicle was not large enough to haul it home. Robert would have no trouble transporting a grill in his "big ol' tank."

We grilled steak, sautéed mushrooms and fixed Tori Lou's favorite potatoes, rubbed with butter and baked in the oven for an hour until crispy on the outside and tender in the middle.

Bread was not included in the menu. I still lacked confidence in my slicing prowess, and had no desire to visit the emergency room again.

Chapter Twenty-Five

My last meeting with Dr. Rossi was Wednesday morning, July 28th, and that evening Tori Lou and I went to my last "Support Group" meeting. I had missed this weekly meeting the previous two times because we were off doing other things. The meetings sometimes did get a little drawn out and I figured Tori Lou would have been a bit bored, so I had waited until my final session to take her along.

As it turned out, we had an excuse for leaving the meeting early. Chris Hamrock, Tori Lou's surfing instructor at Newport Beach, had called a couple of days before and suggested we get together in Chino, where he and Tori Lou could do some skateboarding.

Tori Lou and I were at the meeting long enough for me to tell my fellow proton patients a few things which I felt were important, such as always remembering to spread the word about Loma Linda and proton radiation therapy.

It had become alarmingly obvious to me that a large majority of people across the country, including many highly competent medical professionals, had never even heard of it.

I repeated the story, which I had told at an earlier meeting, about my experience on the shuttle bus at the Ontario airport with the guy who was at Fort Ord the same time as I back in 1967.

Also, I shared with them the way we had resolved to make something bad into something good by taking a positive stance. I urged them never to assume a "woe is me" attitude.

I hoped Tori Lou and I had set an example by taking what could have been a fear-filled, frustrating fight for life and changing it into an often fun-filled, triumphant journey of a lifetime.

"Believe in what you're doing, stay active and upbeat, and tell anyone who'll listen about this special place called Loma Linda," I told the group as they engulfed us with appreciative contemplation while munching their macadamia nut cookies.

"It's not necessary to preach, nor suggest that proton treatment is the only answer, because each man must make his own choice," I said.

"The most important thing is to remind men that forty percent of guys over fifty get this disease and if someone's father or brother has had it, their chances of also getting it are increased."

I added, "If they do find out they have prostate cancer, then proton radiation should be one of the choices they seriously consider."

As Tori Lou stifled a yawn, I continued, "Some men don't even know what a PSA test is or how important check ups are. So, don't be afraid to talk about it and suggest they learn more about what's being done at Loma Linda University Medical Center before making their choice."

The ingrained sense of timing I possessed having once been a disk jockey told me I'd talked long enough without playing a record.

In the midst of polite applause we departed; offering the excuse, "We have an appointment at seven-thirty down in Chino to do some skateboarding."

I added, "This may be the first time somebody left a prostate cancer support group meeting early to go to a skateboard park."

There we a few laughs and some additional polite applause as we hit the hallway, grabbing an extra cookie on the way out.

Chapter Twenty-Six

Chino, a town of about 70,000 people, is just a half hour's drive from Loma Linda. The skate park at Chino is legendary and a lot of Southern California's top skaters hang out there. We weren't surprised to find that Chris Hamrock was as good at skateboarding as he was at surfing.

His board seemed to have jets on it, as he maneuvered the steep curves and walls of the half-pipes and the classic deep bowl with incredible skill. At Chino that night, Tori Lou saw several skaters whom she recognized from skateboard magazines and we met Brett Hamilton, owner of Attic Skateshop in Costa Mesa, and a pretty good skater himself.

Tori Lou was having a blast skating with the "big dogs" at Chino, so we stayed until the park closed. It can get cool at night in Southern California and it was quite chilly in Chino by the time we left. It was the first time in several days we put the top up on the convertible.

Thursday was a busy day; it was the day I would double up on treatments, getting numbers forty-two and forty-three, so I could finish up with number forty-four on Friday, July 30th.

"I ran out of music trivia," I told Tim as I climbed into my pod for my morning treatment, "so here's something different. What was the first product to have a bar code printed on it?"

Always precise in his responses, he answered without a moment's hesitation, "No idea. I can't imagine. How would I know that?"

"Juicy Fruit gum. In 1974." I gave him the answer.

"Oh, yeah. I should have known that," he smiled. "By the way, you're coming back at four-thirty this afternoon, right?"

"Yeah, will you be here?" I asked.

"No, I get off at two. But, I'll be here in the morning for your last one," he assured me.

In the afternoon, when I went back for a second helping of protons, I saw some guys in the changing room I'd never seen before because we were on different schedules.

"Are you a new guy?" one of them asked, "I haven't seen you here before."

"I usually come in during the morning," I explained, "tomorrow's my last treatment."

"Congratulations," he said, "I'm up to number twelve."

"Don't worry; it'll go fast," I assured him.

That was an understatement. I could hardly believe I was almost finished with my proton therapy. In less than twenty-four hours, I would have completed the course to recovery so aptly designed by Dr. Rossi. That's when I started to realize that I would actually miss this place.

Tori Lou spent a good part of the day playing with her friends, Chris and Devon, and visiting Sebastian. I know she was starting to feel as I did about leaving.

While she was anxious to get home to her friends, she, too, would miss this place called Loma Linda, "Where birds sing at night and angels pose as nurses dressed in blue . . ."

Chapter Twenty-Seven

I walked more slowly than usual across the hospital parking lot that Friday morning. I was on my way to Gantry Three for my final proton treatment. As I felt the warm sun on my shoulders and looked up at the San Bernardino Mountains, my thoughts were all over the place. I felt tears starting to materialize, but fought them off. This was indeed a very special place to me and I knew I would miss it.

At the same time I thought of Tori Lou, sleeping soundly in her soft bed, dreaming of getting back with her friends in Wisconsin, and telling them of all the sights she had seen along the way.

I guess we had both become a little spoiled. Tori Lou was having a marvelous time, meeting new friends, seeing new places, learning new skills–her devoted dad tagging along as financier, chauffeur and best friend.

And I had the company of an incredible young daughter, sharing experiences we may never have the chance to do again.

Sure, we would take other trips. I told her I'd

love to take her to Europe and she talked of going on an Alaskan cruise.

"That's the only state you haven't been to, Dad," she'd told me, "and I want to be with you when you go there."

It would not surprise me if, in the near future, she might revise her position on traveling with dad by adding, "If I can bring a friend." Tori Lou was growing up before my eyes and I had to realize that, to her, being with her friends was of top importance. Though she was enjoying the trip, I knew she was anxious to get home; and I would not have her "all to myself" for much longer.

An inner force, of which neither of us was aware at the time, was starting to whisper to her to become more independent. She was on the brink of spreading her wings and testing the flight patterns beyond the nest.

I knew we shared an unbreakable bond and the two of us would always be devoted to one another; but I also knew that this journey had created a special closeness we may never experience again.

Enough of that, I thought, fighting back the

tears. I approached my "secret" entrance to Loma Linda University Medical Center. *I can't let the guys in Gantry Three see me crying,* I thought. Making my way to the changing room, I tried to think ahead to the upcoming eight-day cross country drive back to Wisconsin, which promised to be a memorable part of our journey.

I forgot to bring a trivia question that day, but Tim didn't seem to mind. When the treatment was finished, I thanked the crew and said, "I'll stop in and say, 'hi,' when I come back for my checkup," knowing that I probably would never see some of these guys again.

Back in the changing room, as I was looking in the mirror, untying the perfectly-tied knot behind my neck that held up the hospital gown, the realization that my treatments were actually over hit me. Tears gushed out uncontrollably.

I was never able to establish the predominant source of those tears. Was it relief that the treatments were finished? Was it the knowledge that, maybe, I had finally crushed the chattering cancer gremlins? Or, was it because the whole marvelous journey was almost over?

The best I could determine it was a blend of all of those things. In the mirror I saw my own face, tanned by weeks in the California sun, reflecting a mystifying mosaic of sheer relief, genuine joy and yes . . . profound sadness.

No "discharge" procedure was required for me to leave because, technically, I had been an "outpatient." There we no formalities or paperwork to deal with.

The receptionist, Levita, handed me a plain brown envelope just before I got on the elevator which would take me down one floor, from which I would leave through my secret passageway for the last time.

The envelope contained a certificate of completion from the Brotherhood of the Balloon and a beautiful gold lapel pin with some kind of proton logo that I could never quite figure out. I just knew it represented an accomplishment I should be proud of and for which I should be grateful.

So, that's it? First they told me I was sick. Then they treated me as if I were sick. Then they told me I'm not sick anymore. And, I still feel the same as I did before I found out I had cancer.

It almost seemed too easy. As I walked down my "secret" hallway which would lead me out of the hospital, I contemplated the enormous impact this place has had on so many lives over the years.

Loma Linda Medical Center is a Seventh-Day Adventist Health Sciences Institution, and truly lives up to the Mission Statement posted in the radiation center lobby:

"The mission of Loma Linda University Medical Center is to continue the healing ministry of Jesus Christ, to make man whole, in a setting of advancing medical science and to provide a stimulating clinical and research environment for the education of physicians, nurses, and other health professionals."

Thank God for those who work to advance medical research! As I continued my slow walk out of the medical center, I recalled one of my earliest childhood memories.

I was three years old, playing with toys on the kitchen floor of our home on Tenney Street in Kewanee. I looked up and saw my father, Woodrow, about to go out the front door.

He stood in the foyer, wearing a long black overcoat and a wide-brimmed hat, typical of men's attire in the early 1940's. He appeared older than his thirty years; thin and frail, his skin darkened by the effects of Addison's disease.

At that time, no effective treatment for the ailment was known. I learned, years later, that on that day he was on his way to Mayo Clinic in Rochester, Minnesota to find out if doctors there could do anything to treat his condition.

Something in my little three-year-old heart told me that he was going somewhere special, and I ran to give him a goodbye hug. In my toddler clumsiness, I stumbled and crashed my head squarely into a wooden door case, knocking myself unconscious.

My father died before I had a chance to see him again but I still have a visible scar in the middle of my forehead to remind me of that last vision of my talented dad.

He was a self-taught architect, learning the profession by mail-order schooling. I've often wondered what he might have become, had he lived beyond age thirty. We'll never know.

Today, thanks to research, persons afflicted with Addison's disease can expect to enjoy a normal life expectancy. My father was born too soon to benefit from that research.

Do you think the vision of my dad going out the door crossed my mind, that morning back in May, when I said goodbye to Tori Lou?

You bet it did.

Chapter Twenty-Eight

Tori Lou and I had learned enough about traffic in Southern California to know that leaving on Friday in the middle of the day would be a bad idea. Our plan was to pack up on Friday and then leave early Saturday morning for our drive up to the Hearst Castle.

She spent part of the day Friday playing with her friends, took Sebastian for a walk, and tried to help me figure out how in the world we would get everything in the car.

"We are going to have to ship some of this stuff," Tori Lou proclaimed.

Having anticipated this problem weeks before, I knew the location of the nearest Fed Ex office. We took seven pairs of shoes, one large teddy bear, one blanket given to me by the volunteers, a couple of pairs of long pants, and the optional cover that's designed to put over the convertible top when it's down, and packed all that stuff into two big boxes. Off it went to Wisconsin.

"I'll miss my shoes," Tori Lou said, feigning sadness and wiping a non-existent tear.

"Don't worry," I said, "I insured the stuff for five hundred dollars."

"Can I have the money if they lose it?" she asked, quickly recovering from her despondency, "I could buy a lot of new shoes with five hundred bucks!"

"Forget it," I said. "Fed Ex never loses things. Your shoes will be home before you will."

That evening Tori Lou talked with several friends on her cell phone–friends from Wisconsin and in California. She was saying, "I'll see you soon," to some and "I'll be back to see you again," to others.

"Let's go get Sebastian and take a walk around the campus," I suggested. It was another typically beautiful evening and, so far, no rescue helicopters or emergency vehicles approaching the hospital had broken the stillness.

"Hi, buddy," Tori Lou hollered at Sebastian, who was starting to doze off, probably not expecting to go for a second walk that day. He got up wagging his huge tail, and loped over to his leash, picking it up for Tori Lou. She attached it while he pretended to play a little tug-of-war.

"Let's go," Tori Lou said, and Sebastian looked up with his big, saggy eyes as if to say, "What are we waiting for?"

The three of us strolled the few short blocks to the small, but beautiful campus of Loma Linda University, which had its beginnings early in the twentieth century.

As we walked the campus that evening we marveled at the tall palm trees in the center campus courtyard and at the architecture of some of the older buildings. We wondered if they might be almost 100 years old.

Since being designated, in 1909, by the Seventh Day Adventist Church as a center for educating health professionals, Loma Linda University has grown into one of the premier medical schools in the country. It has sent more of its graduates into international service than any other U.S. medical school.

Loma Linda University Medical Center, with its landmark towers, was opened in 1967 and is recognized as a leader in health-sciences, research and service. Loma Linda University Medical Center became the first hospital-based proton treatment center in 1990.

By spring, 2004 over 9,000 patients had been treated with protons at Loma Linda.

As we strolled beneath the clear California sky that night, the campus area was an enigmatic blend of tranquility and trauma.

Taking a break from our walk, Tori Lou and I relaxed on a park bench in the quiet campus courtyard. Sebastian was in repose next to us, massive nose placed between his huge front paws, contentedly drooling, with all due respect, on the University's nicely manicured lawn.

Just a few hundred yards south of us and seven stories up, a helicopter was approaching, the sound of its blades growing louder as it slowed for its landing. The hospital trauma crew, clothing whipped by the wind from the copter's blades, was at the ready, waiting to receive the incoming patient.

That sight never fails to bring to mind the old adage, "There's always someone worse off than you." I looked down at my thumb; it was healed but still a little tender.

Chapter Twenty-Nine

Saturday, July 31st. Time to leave. I locked the door of the duplex, walked down to the laundry room at the lower level of the building, and put the key in the security drop box where Lorraine could retrieve it later. As Tori Lou and I got in the car, I asked her, "Do you want to go say goodbye to Sebastian?"

"No, that's okay," she said, holding back a tear, "I said goodbye to him last night."

We drove down Barton Road and then headed west on Interstate 10 to begin the more than two thousand mile journey back to Wisconsin.

Wait a minute. West? To Wisconsin? So, there'd be a little back-tracking. We did have eight days!

"Do you have those confirmations we printed out on the computer?" I asked.

"Yep, right here with our maps," yawned Tori Lou. She was still a little tired, having gotten up earlier than she was used to. We had to get to the Hearst Castle by 4:20 P.M. That was the tour time we had reserved online. We'd also reserved a room at the Sea Coast Lodge in San Simeon, but that was a guaranteed reservation, so no worry there. Tori Lou began to wake up a bit as we got further into the greater Los Angeles area.

"Look at that sign, Lou," I said, "Rose Bowl, Next Exit! Did I tell you I went to the Rose Bowl game in 1994, when Wisconsin beat UCLA?"

"One or two hundred times," she said.

She got a little more excited when she saw a green Interstate sign that said, "Hollywood Boulevard" and even more when she spotted the tall building with the sign that said, "Nickelodeon."

Hollywood, Beverly Hills, Burbank, Universal City. Hey, these places really exist! We vowed to come back again when we had some time to spend visiting these places.

The traffic through L.A. was not bad, but once we got on Route 101 things changed. It seemed like half of Los Angeles was heading up the coast for the weekend. It was full-dress, bumper-to-bumper from Oxnard to Santa Barbara, a distance of about sixty miles. While I kept moving my foot on and off the brake pedal, and kept worrying that we might be late for our Hearst Castle tour, Tori Lou slept like a log.

We stopped for lunch in Santa Barbara, a town frequented by celebrities and known for its many great restaurants, such as Rose Café, The Brown Pelican and Stella Mare's. We were in a hurry, so we opted for a time and money saving stop at Jack in the Box. Tori Lou had the Jumbo Jack Burger with Cheese. There was no discussion as to how it ranked along with the burgers at Farmer Boy's and Johnny Rockets. Some mysteries have to be left unsolved.

Once we got north of Santa Barbara, the traffic thinned out and we started moving along the coast at a clip that I knew would get us to the Hearst Castle on time.

Route 101 took us past Vandenberg Air Force Base to San Luis Obispo, where we turned onto California's famous Route One. Around three-thirty P.M. we were in the tiny seaside town of San Simeon, and were approaching the hotel at which we had reserved a room.

We decided to check in later and didn't stop, because it looked like we were going to arrive at Hearst Castle just in time for our tour.

Chapter Thirty

As we neared the entrance to the Hearst Castle Visitors' Center, we saw the pier that was built to handle ships carrying materials and treasures from all over the world, which eventually ended up in the castle we could see off in the distance.

William Randolph Hearst inherited some 250,000 acres of this coastline back in 1919, and commissioned famed San Francisco architect Julia Morgan to "build a little something" for him. By 1947, Hearst and Morgan had created an estate of 165 rooms and 127 acres of gardens, terraces, pools and walkways.

We parked the car and went to the "will call" window to exchange our computer-generated reservation for tickets. The tickets got us immediately on the bus which would take us up the winding road to the castle.

Tori Lou did not want to sit next to the window and had her eyes covered with her hands most of the way. The bus was big; the road was narrow; the hill was steep and there were no guardrails. The woman calmly driving the bus had probably made this trip thousands of times.

"Think of her as an airline pilot," I told Tori Lou.

"Yeah, this is kind of like being in a plane," Tori Lou said. "It's a long way down."

A recorded message played during the trip up the hill and gave some background on the castle. Once our bus had wound its way to the top, a tour guide took us through the 90,000 square foot estate, which includes 56 bedrooms, 41 fireplaces, 61 bathrooms and 19 sitting rooms.

I had been to the Hearst Castle once before, but one could visit dozens of times, and each time see something not seen before. Tori Lou was enamored with the 345,000 gallon swimming pool and the fact that zebras still roamed the area surrounding the castle. William Randolph Hearst had created a menagerie on the premises and some of the animals, or rather their descendents, though seldom seen, still live there.

The drive back down the hill was even more interesting than the drive up. Less than a mile from the visitors' center, our bus broke down. We were stalled just past a curve so traffic coming around the curve would not be able to see us. We feared we might be rear-ended by another bus!

The quick-thinking bus driver, after grumbling for a moment about a "computer glitch," got out and placed flares to warn other drivers. Then, she radioed for help. Within minutes an empty bus pulled alongside and we all transferred into it for the short ride the rest of the way down the hill to the visitors' center.

"So, Tori Lou, did you enjoy it?" I asked.

"The bus ride was kind of scary," she said, "but the castle was awesome!"

So, now they could add the name Victoria Louise Vancil to the Hearst Castle's Guest List, which already included Charlie Chaplin, Clark Gable, Greta Garbo, Winston Churchill, Charles Lindbergh, Amelia Earhart, Harpo Marx, Calvin Coolidge, Louis B. Mayer and William D. Vancil (remember, I had taken the tour once before).

After the tour, we drove back to San Simeon, population 462, and checked in at the Sea Coast Lodge. After carrying our bags up to our room on the second floor, we asked the desk clerk where might be a good place to eat. She recommended the Main Street Grill in Cambria, another small town four miles away.

The food was great, and afterwards we took a short walking tour of Cambria's picturesque Main Street. It featured gift shops, restaurants and real estate offices, as most tourist area towns do. One place in particular caught Tori Lou's eye. It was a small store with a big sign that said, "Vintage Automobilia." It was closed.

"Can we come back here in the morning?" Tori Lou asked. Because of her discussions with Robert McDaniel (the Texan who was our neighbor in Loma Linda) and from looking at Robert's collection of pictures and books, she had become very interested in old cars.

"The sign says the store opens at 10 A.M. and we have to drive all the way to San Francisco tomorrow," I reminded her.

"Well, I won't stay in the store long," she said, "Please, Dad, I think they have some really cool stuff. I could get a book!"

"We'll see," I said.

"OK, let's go back to the hotel," she said. Tori Lou had learned that a "we'll see" from Dad was bankable.

Chapter Thirty-One

Sunday, August 1st, we pulled up in front of the Vintage Automobilia store on Main Street in Cambria exactly at 10 A.M. The store was not open, despite the sign in the window.

"Can we wait for a while?" asked Tori Lou.

"Okay, but not for too long; we have a long drive ahead of us," I answered.

Before checking out of the Sea Coast Lodge in San Simeon, we had enjoyed a complimentary continental breakfast. But Tori Lou suggested we walk across the street to a coffee shop and get a doughnut. I think she was figuring that if I had a hot cup of coffee, it would take some time to finish it; and in the meantime, the Automobilia store would open.

By the time she had eaten her doughnut and I had downed my coffee, it was around 10:30 A.M. and we were both about ready to give up. I knew she was disappointed. We'd wasted quite a bit of time without even entering the store. Just as we were about to get into the car to head for the Big Sur coastline, a truck pulled up with a silver haired man at the wheel.

"That's him," cried Tori Lou, "that's got to be the guy who owns the store!"

She was correct. The store owner, Peter Zobian, called out to us, "Been waiting long?"

"About forty minutes," I said.

"Sorry about that," he replied offering no explanation, "Hope you're not too upset."

"Naw, we're cool. We're from the Midwest," I said, having no idea why I said that, or what it meant.

"Me too, that's why we're all out here," he said. I had no idea what he meant either, but somehow it seemed to make sense at the time.

Once inside the store, I became less concerned about falling behind on our schedule. The "Vintage Automobilia" store was fascinating. Peter had owned the store for over fifty years, we learned, and he was also an antique car collector.

"This is where I start my collection of old car books," Tori Lou said.

I remembered how she'd told Robert McDaniel, back in Loma Linda, that she was interested in books about vintage cars. We asked Peter, the store owner, what he'd recommend. Tori Lou chose an out-of-print book (*Cars, Cars, Cars, Cars* by S.C.H. Davis) which showed pictures and gave information about old cars. It appeared to be a quality book, one that might increase in value over the years.

Seemed like an obvious choice to start a collection. She loved the book, and I was happy she got it. I also knew that, unlike her shoe collection, she would never wear out, nor outgrow, a collection of books.

Peter Zobian's store featured not only books, but vintage toys, posters, old car magazines, and rare parts. I took a picture of Peter and Tori Lou holding a hand-carved crystal hood ornament from a classic car, the name of which I can't remember. But, it had a price tag of over $5,000. (The hood ornament, not the car!)

One wall of the store was covered with photos of hundreds of vintage cars. Each photo was taken, over the years, outside the store in Cambria.

Peter told us that a great-nephew of William Randolph Hearst visits the store from time-to-time, driving up from Los Angeles, to buy vintage toys for his grandchildren.

Before we knew it, it was noon, and we had to get going! Tori Lou climbed into the car with her precious book and donned her white baseball cap, the one with the Hurley logo.

I put on the cool sunglasses I had bought during one of our visits to The Block, donned my green Loma Linda University baseball cap, and off we went. Tori Lou raised her hands above the windshield to feel the fresh, cool ocean air pulsing against her palms and rushing through her fingers.

The sunny drive brought back memories of a hit song I'd played on the radio forty years before. I sang part of the lyrics: "We'll sing in the sunshine . . . we'll laugh every day . . ."

"That was a big hit by Gale Garnett in the Sixties," I explained to Tori Lou. "You probably don't know the song."

"No, I've never heard of him," she said.

"Well, actually, Gale Garnett's a woman," I said.

"Oh, I should have known that," she laughed, mimicking Tim, the technician from Gantry 3, whom I'd told her about.

Chapter Thirty-Two

Sunday, August 1st was a day that we will remember for a long time. We marveled at the sheer, scenic beauty along Route 1, also known as the Pacific Coast Highway. It hugs the coastline called Big Sur and features steep sea cliffs, rugged granite shorelines, redwood forests and cypress trees twisted by the Pacific winds.

Route 1 was completed in 1937, after fifteen years of labor. The many bridges, the most famous of which is the Bixby Creek Bridge, were built in the early years of the project. Anyone who's watched the TV show *"Then Came Bronson"* or has seen the movie *"Brainstorm"* (Natalie Wood's last film) would recognize the majestic, arched, Bixby Creek Bridge.

We stopped many times to take pictures. At one of the "scenic view" rest stops, Tori Lou spotted an unexpected bonus; a four-wheeled "scenic beauty"–a silver and black 1955 Ford Thunderbird convertible!

"Did I ever tell you I used to own a '57 T-Bird, Lou?" I asked.

"Only about 200 times," she reminded me, "it

was white, right? With the little portholes in the side?"

"Black and white leather interior," I mumbled.

As we walked over to peek inside the car, a man and his teenage son were walking toward us.

"Is this your car?" I asked, "Do you mind if we take a picture of it? My daughter collects pictures of classic cars."

I didn't tell him the collection had just started that day and all the pictures were in one book. You have to start somewhere.

"I've got a better idea," the car owner said, "why don't I take a picture of the two of you standing next to the car?"

Wow! Not only are we getting a picture of the car, but a picture of us and the car . . . taken by the owner. That's water-cooler talk for sure.

We talked with the T-Bird owner and his son for a few minutes and learned that he was from Hong Kong. He owns property in Southern California and in Oregon and they were taking the car from California to their property in the Great Northwest.

He said he's an importer, and had been in Wisconsin recently, doing business with a large multi-location, retail, home-improvement chain that is headquartered in the state.

"Oh, the place with the piercing TV commercials that drive me nuts," I said. The man's blank look suggested he'd not seen those commercials. Lucky for him, he'd never *heard* them either.

There, in that tranquil place beside the sea, for just a moment, I could hear the earsplitting voice of that commercial announcer echoing off the granite cliffs.

"Some things you just can't get away from," I thought. I put my hands over my ears and staged a muted scream.

The drive along the Big Sur was breathtaking. Tori Lou and I were both glad we had changed the original itinerary for the route home. Our plan was to drive the 100 mile stretch from San Simeon to Monterey on Route 1, and then get back on Route 101, a faster way to make it into San Francisco.

We'd hoped to get there before dark. Our plan would have worked, except there was a traffic accident on 101 ahead of us, near Monterey, so it ended up taking us longer to get to San Francisco than if we had stayed on the narrower, more winding coastal route. But, Route 101 did give us the opportunity to drive past Fort Ord, the Army base where I was stationed almost forty years before. I remembered the shuttle bus driver, whom I tipped off about Loma Linda back in March.

Fort Ord was closed in 1994, after it had been used as a training facility off and on since 1846. The base is still used for a variety of purposes, mostly non-military and the buildings we saw from the freeway looked as sturdy and as well-cared-for as they did back in 1967.

Some intimidating memories of Fort Ord flashed through my mind as we drove past the barbed wire fences that surround the property. Completing AIT (Advance Infantry Training) was a physical and mental challenge.

I remembered being rousted out of bed at four A.M., well before dawn, and running six or seven miles out into the foothills with full battle gear - steel helmet, backpack, M-16 rifle, big heavy boots and thick rubber poncho.

Out in the foothills our squadron sat in bleachers, a sort of outdoor classroom, while the chilly March wind off the Pacific snuck inside our ponchos and almost froze our sweating bodies. After an hour of shivering through class, learning how to set up a mortar or dig a latrine, we'd run in cadence back to the barracks and have breakfast, clean up our gear and get ready for an inspection.

I didn't share all the torturous memories with Tori Lou. It was nearly impossible to come up with anything fun to tell about Fort Ord, but I did think of one thing. It was the cadence that we chanted, as we marched or ran in unison.

"You had a good home, but you left!" the drill sergeant would shout.

"You're right!" my fellow trainees and I would shout back, as our right feet pummeled the ground. And so it went, over and over.

"You had a good home, but you left!" . . ."You're right!" "You had a good home, but you left!" (pause) "Jody was there when you left" . . ."You're right." "Jody was there when you left. . . ."

Tori Lou joined me in mimicking the Army marching chant and we continued it for a few minutes, laughing throughout. It was a way to break the monotony of the slowed down traffic situation in which we found ourselves.

"Who was Jody, Dad?" Tori Lou asked.

"Ahh . . . Jody is the guy back home who, at least in the soldier's imagination, is trying to court his girlfriend . . . while he's away with the Army," I explained as best I could.

"Oh, I think I saw something about that on TV," she answered.

Chapter Thirty-Three

"Hey, look! San Francisco–'Left Three Lanes,'" Tori Lou said excitedly, pointing at the highway sign. "Move over one lane, Dad."

In the not-too-far distance we could see some ominous clouds piled high like gray, triple-dip ice cream cones. They were surrounded by a wandering, foggy haze that looked chilly and damp.

"Yeah, that's San Francisco," I said, as we pulled over to put the convertible top up.

The rain was light, and so was the traffic, as we drove the Bayshore Freeway along San Francisco Bay, passed the airport, and 3COM Park (formerly Candlestick Park) and wound our way into the heart of the city. We had a reservation at the Holiday Inn Select, next to the famous Triangle Building, and a block from Chinatown. We checked into the hotel, parked in the ramp, and carried our bags to the elevator that took us to our room on the twenty-sixth floor.

The sun was just beginning to set, when we entered the room and pulled open the blinds to see what sort of view we had. We were looking north and dead center in front of us was Coit Tower, sitting majestically atop Telegraph Hill.

The tower was built in 1933 as a memorial to San Francisco's firefighters who fought the fires during the earthquake in 1906. Some people say that the tower looks like a fire hose nozzle.

"Look, Dad, there's Alcatraz!" said Tori Lou, "I thought it would be bigger."

"It *is* big. It's just far away," I pointed out. "Remember how much smaller the Hearst Castle looked from a distance?"

"And, I remember that when you get closer to the mountains, they get easier to see," she said.

"Are you getting hungry?" I asked, knowing what the answer would be.

The last time we'd eaten was at an isolated, roadside restaurant tucked into the side of a cliff somewhere along the Pacific Coast Highway. The bill was twelve dollars for two hot dogs, two cans of soda and a bag of potato chips. Location is all-important in the restaurant business.

That theory was proven wrong when, on the evening of our arrival in San Francisco, we ate dinner at an Italian Restaurant located in the first block of Chinatown. The Mona Lisa Restaurant was recommended by the hotel concierge, and it was just three blocks from the hotel, so we walked there.

The restaurant was full, but there were a couple of small round tables available in front, along the sidewalk. The sun had gone down and it was getting chilly, but we decided to sit outside. It would be fun. The restaurant had set up overhead gas heaters which warmed the area, so it was quite comfortable.

The food was excellent. Tori Lou ordered fettuccini alfredo and I decided on calamari.

"Dad, that's squid!" Tori Lou pointed out.

"I know; it's great deep fried. They have really good calamari here in California," I said. "I'll let you try some."

The waiter brought out a basket of bread and a bottle of garlic dipping oil. As I picked up one of the pieces of bread, I glanced at my thumb and thought, "I'm glad this is already sliced."

Unable to deny curiosity, Tori Lou actually tasted the calamari and, much to my surprise, seemed to like it. "Pretty good," she said. "Tastes like chicken."

"It does, sort of. Want some more?" I asked.

"No, I'm okay," she said, scooping up some of her fettuccini.

Instinct told me that when a thirteen-year-old tastes calamari and says, "Pretty good," and then declines a second bite, it really means, "Now you know what unconditional love is, but one bite of calamari is enough."

After dinner, we walked back to our hotel, stopping to browse in a couple of gift shops and a book store along the way. Tori Lou couldn't find any good "old car books;" it wasn't that kind of store. It featured books about medieval political philosophy and postmodernism, works by Wharton, Heller, Kerouac and Freud. Not a single book about vintage cars.

Luckily, we had our digital camera along, because as we were getting near the front entrance of the hotel, Tori Lou exclaimed, "Dad, look! Parked over there, right in front of the hotel! It's a Jaguar XJS!"

This kid knew her cars! She took the picture, and then walked closer, for a better look. "It's a V-12! Twelve cylinders! Wow!" she said.

Our first night in San Francisco, we fell asleep fairly easily. It had been a busy day.

As we dozed off, the light from the rotating beacon on Alcatraz Island moved silently and hauntingly across our hotel room wall.

Chapter Thirty-Four

It was August 2nd, two months and a day since I walked into Gantry Three at Loma Linda Medical Center to begin proton treatment. I remembered how I lay in the pod that first day thinking, "Forty-three more to go."

Not once did I say, or even think, "This is going to take a long time." Within myself, I knew time would pass all too quickly.

I had been asked by friends, "Won't you be glad when this is over and you can go home and get back to your normal routine?"

"No, why would I want it to be over?" I answered, "I'm enjoying this adventure; and when the treatments are finished, three more months of my life will have passed."

When you're a kid, you think you are going to live forever. When you get a bit older, you start to realize you're not. And, when you get cancer, you become certain of it. The matter of time becomes paramount. Every day becomes more precious. Life-altering experience? You bet.

Over the centuries, man has invented ways to measure and save this precious thing called time.

In 1876, Seth Thomas introduced the wind-up alarm clock, so people could wake up and make the most of each day. In 1953 Carl Swanson invented the TV dinner, so we could watch Ed Sullivan and eat previously frozen food at the same time.

Woody Allen is sometimes given credit for the quote, "Time is nature's way of keeping everything from happening at once." Others give credit to "anonymous." Regardless, I've quoted that line often. Time does tend to spread things out, but as you get older, events and the spaces between them become more compacted.

So, here I was, in San Francisco, looking out the window at the fog-shrouded city awakening to start its Monday morning routine. I thought of how quickly we move through stages of life, as I gazed at my beautiful daughter, still sleeping.

I thought, "Some day, my Victoria Louise will grow old." I tried to visualize her as an old lady and just couldn't imagine. If only I had the power to look into the future. What horizons will she cross? What triumphs will she enjoy? With her many talents, she has every opportunity to live a full and happy life.

Perhaps an omen of things to come for this accomplished skateboarder and vintage-car buff, she walked before she was eight months old and her first three-syllable word was "Cadillac."

My hope was that this trip would be an inspiration to her to continue to learn and grow and to appreciate the value of staying well.

I also hoped that she would keep the attitude we had grown to share, *"Don't fear the big dogs."*

This "motto," obviously, doesn't apply to vicious attack dogs, of either the canine or humanoid variety. What it means is, "Don't be afraid to speak your mind, stand up for what's fair, enter competition with an attitude of doing your best, be active instead of passive when there's something important at stake.

The motto can be applied in many situations.

For a kid, it can be as simple as walking up to a 160 pound Great Dane and gaining his friendship with a kind word and a pat on the head, or entering a skateboard competition when all the other contestants are boys and you're a girl. It can mean putting your hand up in class and sharing your thoughts, even though a bully might tease you about it in the hall later.

For an adult, it can mean standing up to a store manager and demanding a refund for poor service or for a product with which you were disappointed, telling your doctor you want a second opinion, standing up in front of a board of directors and suggesting that one of their policies needs revision.

Or, it can mean facing a life-threatening disease in a pro-active way, showing determination and a positive attitude.

"Don't fear the big dogs," means having confidence in yourself, your abilities and your resolve; and it means not being afraid to apply that attitude in an appropriate manner, in any situation, with any sort of person.

Now, it was time to awaken my skater / surfer / artist / musician / analyst daughter and get on with the business of spending some precious time having fun. And, what better place to do it than the "City by the Bay"?

Chapter Thirty-Five

We looked forward to having the entire day to spend in San Francisco, and to one more night watching the Alcatraz beacon trace the wall of our hotel room. This would be the first time, since we'd been together in California that we wouldn't get in the car, at all, for an entire day. The Spyder would get a well-deserved rest in the safe confines of the hotel parking ramp. We studied the map of the downtown area and decided the best way to see the city was on foot and by cable car.

Before we left the hotel room I said, "Let's make sure we have everything we need, Lou. You got the digital camera?"

"It's there on the dresser," she answered, as she picked it up. "Can I carry it, in case I see any cool cars?"

"Sure," I said, "do you have one of the room keys, just in case we get separated?" As if I would ever let her out of my sight.

"Yep, right here," she answered.

"It might get chilly if we stay out past dark, and you didn't bring a jacket, did you?" Our original plan had been to stay in Southern California and not venture into the naturally cooler Bay Area.

"I'll buy a hoody that says San Francisco!" she proclaimed. (A "hoody" is skateboard talk for hooded sweatshirt.) "They have some cool stores at Pier 39 don't they?"

It was obvious she had done her homework and was well aware that there were a ton of stores at Pier 39.

"Do you have your reading glasses, Dad?" Tori Lou asked.

"Right here," I said.

"Map? Cell phone?" she asked.

"Yep," I said.

"Credit card?" she smiled.

"Now, what would we need that for?" I asked.

"Let's go, Dad" she said, heading toward the door. "We're wasting time. Do you think we could tour Alcatraz?"

As we were going down in the elevator, I told her, "I think you have to make reservations something like three weeks ahead of time to tour Alcatraz."

I had looked into this previously, and knew advance reservations we're required, but added, "We'll check to make sure."

Our first stop was at a coffee shop, not far from the restaurant where we had dined the night before. Tori Lou had her traditional bagel with peanut butter (special order). I had one with cream cheese, and a cup of coffee.

Between bites, Tori Lou and I looked at the map and planned our itinerary. We decided to walk up Columbus Avenue, through China-town, and then take Stockton Street, through North Beach, to Fisherman's Wharf and Pier 39. After visiting the pier, we would head West toward Ghiradelli Square, and see how far our energy would take us. Then we'd return to our hotel, riding a cable car at least part of the way back. We knew there was a big choice of restaurants within walking distance of the hotel, so we'd have no trouble finding a place to have dinner that evening.

As we strolled amidst the hustle and bustle of Chinatown, we crossed San Francisco's oldest street, Grant Avenue. This street, immortalized in the musical, "Flower Drum Song," runs eight blocks through the center of Chinatown. We took pictures of some of the pagoda-roofed buildings and storefronts and Tori Lou captured a nice photo of an old Alfa Romeo roadster.

"So, Lou, last night we ate at an Italian restaurant in Chinatown and now you're here taking pictures of an Italian car," I kidded.

"It's okay, Dad," she explained as if she were a young international diplomat, "we'll have Chinese for dinner tonight."

After a few blocks, as we were leaving Chinatown and entering the North Beach area, we noticed something different about the traffic lights at some intersections. Along with the standard "Walk" or "Don't Walk" signal for pedestrians, there was also a "countdown clock" that counted down the seconds . . . 9–8-7–6-5–4-3–2-1. At zero it would change to "Don't Walk."

At the next intersection, we quickly learned that this was a new device, recently installed in San Francisco. A television newsman with microphone in hand, and another man with a camera, approached us, as we were about to cross the street.

"We're from KCBS-TV, could we get your opinion on something?" the newsman asked.

"Sure," I replied, recognizing an opportunity for instant stardom.

"What do you think of the new pedestrian countdown lights?" he asked.

"This is the first time we've seen them," I said. "I guess it's a good idea."

Knowing this was not a very provocative answer and would probably end up on the cutting room floor, I added, "But, what happens when it gets to zero and some slow person is still in the middle of the street?"

"Well, that's the controversy," explained the newsman, "some people think motorists will be looking at the light and paying attention to it, rather than watching for pedestrians."

I can't remember what else either of us said, but I think the newsman and I both realized this interview wasn't going anywhere and it was probably a "non-story" anyway; so he thanked us and we proceeded on our way.

As we continued north toward Fisherman's Wharf, Tori Lou hit the jackpot, getting pictures of an orange-colored, vintage BMW and a '65 Ford Mustang. Her collection of old car photos was growing quickly.

As we approached Fisherman's Wharf, Tori Lou spotted a big sign that read, "Alcatraz Tours."

"Let's see if maybe we can go," she said.

My earlier research turned out to be correct. As we approached the ticket booth, we saw the notice posted. It would be three weeks before we could get on one of the tours.

"I don't think we want to wait that long, do you?" I asked.

"Probably not," she winced, "It's okay; we'll do the tour next time we're here."

I hope we get that chance sometime. It is impossible to properly tour San Francisco in a day-and-a-half.

It didn't take long for her to recover from the mild disappointment. We reached Pier 39, a mecca for tourists and home to over a hundred shops and restaurants. It's one of the most visited tourist spots in America.

She found the hooded sweatshirt she'd wanted in one of the first stores we visited. It zipped up the front and said "San Francisco." It was perfectly understated fashion for a cool evening in the city, or to wear skateboarding back home in Wisconsin.

From the pier we had our closest view of Alcatraz; and saw the famous sea lions that bark at the tourists, bask in the sun and generally show off just a few feet from the edge of the pier.

We had lunch at one of the many restaurants and then stopped in a "make-your-own-candle" studio called "Waxen Moon."

We decided to give it a try. The procedure was simple, the outcome terrific. We cut small chunks of wax, choosing from a variety of colors, and placed them in a mold made of tin. There was a wick suspended vertically in the center.

After we filled the molds, the store owner, Candy, poured hot liquid wax into the mold to fill in all the gaps and crevices. She told us to come back in about twenty minutes to pick up the candles, which needed time to cool. Tori Lou said she was going to give the one she made to her mom, as a souvenir.

As we walked along, waiting for our candles, I recalled other projects Tori Lou and I had worked on together in the past, some for school, and others just for fun. Some involved painting or building with wood and cardboard, others required cutting and pasting pictures from magazines; and more recently, searching for information on the internet. The "cutting and pasting" has become less messy. It's done on the computer.

With each project, I've seen her artistic talent coming through more and more. By the time she was ten years old she was proficient with the computer graphics program I use for designing websites professionally. She has discovered how to do things with the program that I hadn't been aware of.

I recalled the time when she was doing a project on the computer. She had asked me how to spell a word that contained the letter "o." Instead of spelling it out verbally, I just reached over and typed in the word for her.

She looked at the word, then looked up at me and said, "Dad, an 'o' is a circle and a 'zero' is an oval, except in some fonts." Clearly, I'd hit the wrong key.

"And I found an easier way to put in a graduated fountain fill," she added.

More than once, I'd joked to friends, "It's amazing how far we've come. Kids in elementary school are using computers! When Abe Lincoln and I were in school, back in Illinois, we did our homework on the back of a wooden shovel with a piece of coal."

After we picked up our candles, which both looked great, once they'd cooled and been removed from the molds, we continued our exploration of the waterfront.

We came across a couple of "living statues," guys who had completely sprayed themselves and their clothing using cans of silver paint. They stood motionless holding a cup, until someone put a dollar in the cup. Then the "statue" would come to life, showing gradual movement that evolved into a slow-motion moon walk, before suddenly freezing again, in a pose designed to evoke more contributions.

"Interesting way to make a living," I thought.

The next "statues" we saw didn't move, but were quite intriguing nevertheless.

"Wax Museum!" Tori Lou exclaimed, pointing across the street, "Can we go?"

"Sure," I said, "Why not?" I was a real "soft touch" that day.

Inside the Wax Museum, Tori Lou asked me to take pictures of her, standing in front of her favorites; Beetlejuice, Rambo, and Scarface.

And then she took one picture of me, standing in front of my old schoolmate, Abraham Lincoln.

We were getting tired and decided to head back toward our hotel. We walked to the cable car turnaround at the corner of Taylor and Bay.

There was a long line waiting to board, but we decided it would be worth the wait. How could we visit San Francisco without riding a cable car?

There was a guy sitting on a folding chair playing tenor saxophone and sometimes singing. He was pretty good on the sax, not so good on the singing. But, he had collected a fair number of contributions, tossed into his sax case by tourists waiting to ride the cable cars.

Finally, it was our turn to climb onto one of the cable cars. As the cable started pulling up the hill, the music of the saxophone faded into the distance and was soon drowned out by the clanking of the cable pulling beneath the car.

The car was crowded, but we enjoyed watching the passing sights, as it clanked its way up Columbus to Mason Street, and then took a hard left onto Washington. After one block, we were at the corner of Powell Street, where we pulled the cord to signal the driver to let us off.

We were right back in the heart of Chinatown and just a few blocks from our hotel. The day had gone quickly; we'd done a lot and we were in need of a rest. We stopped at an ice cream shop and each got a cone, then sat at a small table, just outside the shop, and took a break before walking the remaining block or so back to the hotel.

After resting in our room for awhile, we decided to find a place to have dinner. The night before, the concierge had directed us to an Italian restaurant and the food was great; so we decided to ask him again.

"We like that restaurant you suggested last night," I said to the concierge.

"But, tonight we want to have Chinese," Tori Lou added.

We thought he might suggest something with an exotic sounding oriental name like "Imperial Pagoda" or "Shanghai Dragon" right in the heart of Chinatown.

"I think the best place around for Chinese," he said, "is R & G Lounge just up here on Kearney Street, right near the edge of "Little Italy."

So, we were headed for a Chinese restaurant on the edge of Little Italy (after dining the night before in an Italian Restaurant on the edge of Chinatown). At the place with the unlikely name R & G Lounge, we had the best Chinese food either of us had ever eaten.

Later we learned that this place was a favorite of local residents and tourists who had been lucky enough to discover it amidst all the other places with more exotic names.

After dinner, we stopped in a souvenir shop, which featured about ten million baseball caps with inscriptions stating everything from "Property of Alcatraz" to "Green Bay Packers."

Finally, we made it back to our hotel. Under the unwavering watch of the beacon from the Big House, we fell asleep quickly.

Chapter Thirty-Six

Tuesday, August 3rd, we checked out of the Holiday Inn Select, packed up the car and pulled out onto Kearney Street. Our plan was to reach Reno, Nevada and spend the night there.

"Reno's not that far," I said to Tori Lou, "It probably won't take us more than three or four hours to get there."

"Should we see a little more of San Francisco before we leave town?" I asked.

"Sure, this place is really cool," she replied, "can we drive down the crookedest street in the world?"

A quick look at the map showed that the section of Lombard Street she was referring to was only a few blocks away, in the Russian Hill neighborhood.

We found the street, abounding with Victorian mansions and colorful flower beds. This area is home to some of the most expensive real estate in the country. I carefully inched the car down the series of hairpin turns. Though no speed limit was posted, it was obvious that anything over 2 miles per hour would be risky.

At the bottom of the block long hill, several tourists were taking pictures of the street from the bottom up. "Did you know there's a street in Burlington, Iowa that claims to be more crooked than this one?"

"I'm hungry," was her response, "we haven't had breakfast."

"There's a restaurant called the Cliff House that is famous for waffles," I told her, "but, it's pretty far; clear out at the beach, probably six or seven miles. Right near the Cliff House are the Seal Rocks, little islands close to the shore which are usually covered with seals."
"Let's go. We have plenty of time to get to Reno," she said, "plus, we'll get to see the ocean one more time before we head home."

Neither of us was all that anxious to leave this fascinating city. We turned onto Geary Street and headed west, hoping we would not have to wait in line at the Cliff House for breakfast.

Geary Street is a very straight street and one of the longest in the city. We were on Geary for about seventy-five blocks and then veered off onto Point Lobos Avenue, which took us to the spot where the Cliff House is located, right on the ocean.

To our disappointment, we discovered that the Cliff House was closed, undergoing extensive remodeling. So, without stopping, we turned onto Great Avenue, a scenic drive that hugs the beach for miles along the Pacific Ocean. We pulled over and parked the car, to get a view of the ocean and have a good look at the Seal Rocks. To our dismay, not only had we found the Cliff House closed, but there were no seals to be seen anywhere!

"Oh, well. We'll come here again, when we come back to visit Alcatraz," Tori Lou rationalized. "At least we got to see the ocean again. It's the ocean where I learned to surf!"

I couldn't resist boring Tori Lou with another ancient anecdote.

"You know, Lou. This is the same ocean in which I learned to water ski," I said matter-of-factly.

"No way!" she declared, "you learned to water ski in an ocean?" She thought water skiing was a Wisconsin lake thing.

"It was 1957," I told her, "I was sixteen."

"Did you have a driver's license?" she asked.

"Yes, but Frank did all the driving," I said, trying to keep the anecdote on track. "We drove to Houston then took a bus all the way to Acapulco. Remember, my stepfather wouldn't fly."

"What kind of car did you have?" she asked.

"Well, it was about a '56 Buick," I guessed.

"No, what kind of car did *you* have," she persisted, "Didn't you have your own car when you were sixteen?"
"Actually, I don't think I got my own car until the next year, when I was seventeen," I said.

I couldn't remember for sure, but didn't want Tori Lou to think that every kid automatically gets a car along with getting their license. "It was a '49 Ford," I added.

"Sweet!" she said.

"So, do you want to hear about how I learned to water ski?" I asked.

"I guess," she said, while peering through

our binoculars, "Those rocks are covered with white stuff. Is that the color of the rock, or do the seals go to the bathroom a lot on them?"

Now that it was clear that I had her complete attention, I continued my story. "Minnie, Frank and I were on a beach in Acapulco, where they have what's called the "Morning Beach" and the "Afternoon Beach."

We were on the "Morning Beach" when a man and woman, both extremely tan and friendly asked, "Would you be interested in water ski lessons?" They had no accents; they had probably moved here from Michigan or somewhere.

"Hey, Mom, can I?" I pleaded. I was a small, male, 1957 version of Tori Lou.

"How much is it?" Frank and Minnie asked in unison.

"Five dollars for two hours," the boat owner responded.

Five dollars was one forty-fifth of what I would pay for Tori Lou's surfing lesson two score and seven years later, but at the time it seemed like a sizable investment.

I got my way, and off I went with two strangers in their ski boat, to learn something I'd never done before. There was no *"fearing the big dogs"* that day.

As we were getting into the boat, they announced, "We'll go around the peninsula to the "Afternoon Beach;" the water's smoother over there.

After a fifteen minute ride out into the ocean and around the peninsula, we finally slowed down and stopped in the shallows a few yards off the "Afternoon Beach." I climbed out of the boat and into the water with the man and he helped me get into the skis.

Handing me the tow rope, he said, "Now, hold your arms straight and don't let go!" he shouted from the boat.

He hit the gas and the boat took off like a rocket, popping me out of the skis immediately.

Remembering the advice, "Don't let go," I held on for dear life. Only one thing wrong; I was underwater with no skis, hanging on to the tow rope and traveling beneath the surface at a speed that would have made Flipper take notice.

After about ten seconds, I realized this was not right; so I let go and popped to the surface.

"We forgot to tell you to point your skis up, out of the water," they explained.

On the next try, I did what I was told, got almost all the way up, but fell over after a few seconds. Third try was a charm; I made it up and was skiing along atop the water with a shaky kind of confidence.

After it became apparent, to the duo on the boat, that I had my balance and was doing pretty well, they shouted, "We are heading back to the 'Morning Beach;' your two hours are almost up. Just hang on."

With those words, they headed the boat back out into the open sea to make the return, round-about trip back to the other beach. As we got further out from shore, perhaps a quarter of a mile or so, I began to experience a bit of a panic attack.

I was doing okay with the skiing; wobbly, but still up and running. However, being out that far from shore rattled my nerves.

"Sharks!" I thought. "I know these have to be shark-infested waters. If I fall down, I'm dead.

Please, God, let me stay above the water. Please, boat, go fast enough the sharks can't catch us."

I was so scared, I started shaking and the rope became a little slack. I lost my balance and down I went!

"Yikes! I'm a goner," I thought, holding the ski upright so the rescue boat could spot me and pull me to safety, if it wasn't already too late. I kept watching for steel-blue fins cutting through the warm water in which I was floating.

"You did great!" said the woman, as the guy pulled me into the boat.

"Thanks," I said, trying to act as though I'd cheated death many times before and thought nothing of it.

As I finished telling my Acapulco water-skiing story, Tori Lou and I continued to look at the ocean from our spot along the Esplanade. There were actually a few surfers in wet suits braving the cold water.

"It looks a lot colder here than at Newport Beach," she said. "But, I would try it, if I had a wet suit." I knew she was correct on both counts.

Neither of us was anxious to drive away from this spot. It was the farthest West we would venture on our journey; leaving it symbolized the beginning of the end of our trip.

Chapter Thirty-Seven

While heading East on Geary Boulevard back toward the city, we decided to take a short side trip. Since we were in the neighborhood, why not see another of the city's great attractions? We turned left on 34th Avenue and found the entrance to Lincoln Park, then wound our way through the park golf course to the Palace of the Legion of Honor. It is San Francisco's most beautiful museum, with an impressive collection of Ancient and European art.

As we walked through the outdoor Court of Honor, Tori Lou recognized Rodin's best known work, the Thinker, one of more than seventy Rodin sculptures housed in the museum, along with one of the largest collections of prints and drawings in the country. The building was completed in 1924, and was built to honor the 3,600 California men who died in France, during World War I.

Although we had experienced bad fortune in attempting to visit the Cliff House, our luck was quite the opposite at the Legion of Honor.

Three days earlier, internationally known Austrian artist Gottfried Helnwein had opened his first one-man museum exhibition in the United States, "The Child: Works by Gottfried Helnwien" consisted of over fifty paintings, drawings, watercolors, and photographs spanning the period from the early 1970s, until the present.

On top of that, it happened to be a Tuesday, when admission was free, courtesy of Ford Motor Company. Every once in a while, something happens to prove the truth in the old saying, "The best things in life are free."

We found our way through the city and got onto Interstate 80, which would ultimately take us across almost two-thirds of America. For our first day on I-80, however, our goal was just to get to "The Biggest Little City in the World." Our first step toward Reno, Nevada, was to cross the San Francisco–Oakland Bay Bridge, an engineering marvel. The Bay Bridge, which is actually two bridges connected by a tunnel that goes under Yerba Buena Island, carries an average of over a quarter-of-a-million vehicles a day.

After driving the eight-and-a-half miles across the Bay Bridge, we found ourselves in Oakland; and, for the first time on our trip, we were lost. We had been on Interstate 80 for less than twenty minutes and all of a sudden, we weren't on it anymore. We'd missed one of those green signs somewhere and were totally lost, somewhere in Oakland. So, we did the only sensible thing to do under the circumstances. We stopped for lunch.

"Burger King. Right there, Dad," said Tori Lou, pointing at the first fast food place we came across. We took our California roadmap inside with us to try and figure out how to get back on track. As we ate our Junior Whoppers and fries, we studied the map. "Right here is where we must have been in the wrong lane, Dad," explained Tori Lou.

"It's really easy to miss a turnoff, you know," she counseled, "and sometimes when it says merge, you don't really merge, you just . . ." Then, interrupting herself, she said, "Why don't we ask those guys over there."

Three men, who appeared to be construction workers on lunch break, were happy to help us out. "Just go down this street for about five blocks and take a left; you'll see a sign to Interstate 80."

As we headed out of Oakland, passing through Vallejo and skirting the wine country near Napa, Tori Lou was studying the map.

"When we get to Sacramento, we'll be almost

halfway to Reno," she explained. "It's the state capital, isn't it?"

"No, Carson City's the capital, but it's real close to Reno," I answered.

"I didn't mean Nevada," Tori Lou replied, "I meant Sacramento. Is it the capital of California?"

"Yes, it is," I said, "but, we won't see much of it."

"If you just go through a place, can you say you've been there?" she asked.

"I suppose," I said, wondering where she was going with that.

"Good. Because, by the time we get home we will have been in six state capitals in five days!" she explained, slapping her thigh with the map.

"Without ever getting on a plane," I smiled. By now she knew the routine about my step-father, Frank, never wanting to fly.

"Sacramento, Salt Lake City, Cheyenne, Lincoln, Des Moines and Madison," she counted them off. "Too bad Reno's not the capital of Nevada."

"Did I ever tell you about the one and only time my step-dad, Frank, did fly?" I asked her.

"You said he never flew," she stated.

"Well, he didn't fly at all during those trips around the country and to Europe," I clarified, "but, there was one time when he finally did get on a plane. It was 1957, the year after our trip to Europe. We had driven all the way from Kewanee, Illinois to Houston and then took a bus to Acapulco."

"Where you learned to water ski?" she remembered.

"Right," I continued, "well, the bus ride to Acapulco from Houston took about forty hours and the bus was not air conditioned."

"Were there chickens on the bus?" she asked, apparently having seen that on TV or in a movie.

"There might have been," I said, "I know it was such a terrible ride, it convinced Frank to fly back to Houston where we had left the car!"

"So, how was the flight?" Tori Lou asked.

"Not as bad as the bus ride, but pretty bad," I said. "We boarded the plane in the evening and it was dark. The flight attendant (at that time they were called stewardesses) showed us on to the plane with a flashlight."

"We can't turn on the lights inside the plane until the engines have been started," she explained. "They are run by generators which are part of the engines."

I had never seen my stepfather frightened before, and I was a little shaky myself, because this was to be my first airplane flight also. Come to think of it, it may have been the first for my mother, as well.

At any rate, we arrived safely in Houston and Frank never, ever flew again. He also never took another bus to Mexico."

Chapter Thirty-Eight

East of Sacramento we started gaining elevation, driving into the Sierra Nevada Mountains. It was still Tuesday, and hard to believe that we'd seen so much in just half a day. Hours earlier we were gazing out at the Pacific Ocean, and now we were approaching Donner Pass, the infamous "shortcut" through the Sierras where, over 150 years before, a wagon train was stranded by winter weather and many emigrants starved to death. It was perhaps the most famous story of tragedy to come out of the Westward Movement.

But it was during August at Donner Pass, the Tuesday we were there, and the weather was beautiful. We pulled into a rest stop, nestled in a beautiful setting with tall trees stretching toward the blue sky and huge boulders resting innocently behind the visitor's building. A stone monument documented the story of the Donner wagon train party and their fate back in the winter of 1846–47.

"Hey, Dad, give me the digital camera!" shouted Tori Lou as she pointed to a car sitting at the far end of the parking area. "It's a '57 Chevy!"

"There are some people in the car," I cautioned, "You'd better ask them if it's okay."

After Tori Lou got permission and had taken a couple of pictures of the two-tone white and aqua Chevy, we chatted with the owners for a minute.

"If you like cars, you should be headed to Reno," they told us.

"We are. What's going on in Reno?" Tori Lou asked.

"It's called 'Hot August Nights,'" they explained, "It's just getting started and will run all week. There will be hundreds of show cars and the Beach Boys and . . ." Tori Lou's eyes lit up. This was some gift from above, for sure. Imagine! "Hot August Nights!" And we are going to be there!

"You might have trouble finding a hotel room," the owner of the '57 Chevy told us. "The place will be packed."

I suspected that Reno was the type of town that never runs out of hotel rooms; but to be safe, we called ahead. Using the cell phone, I made a reservation at Circus Circus. Within a couple of hours we descended the Eastern slope of the Sierra Nevadas and were pulling into Reno.

As we checked into Circus Circus Hotel, we overheard some people talking about "Hot August Nights." They were saying that there would be thousands of classic cars in town for this huge event and, come evening, all those in town so far would be "cruising" the main drag. Tori Lou could hardly wait.

We had dinner in one of the hotel restaurants and then visited the Circus Circus arcade. Tori Lou loved playing the games that printed out tickets which could be redeemed for prizes. In the main showroom, above the arcade, a troop of trapeze artists entertained.

After spending about an hour in the arcade (and spending about as much money as I might have lost had I gone into the casino) we decided to go looking for cars to photograph.

It's no wonder "Hot August Nights" has become such a popular annual event. Hundreds of shined-up show cars cruise the main drag, with the neon lights of the hotels, casinos and shops as a backdrop. It's a motorized, magical scene.

We stationed ourselves near the intersection of Virginia Street and Commercial Row, where one of the most photographed tourist attractions in the country stands; its famous lighted arch that reads "Reno–The Biggest Little City in the World."

"I'll stand right here at the stop light," directed Tori Lou, "and when a cool car stops I will take pictures. If we're not sure what kind of car it is or what year, you ask them? Okay?"

"Sure, but we didn't bring anything to take notes," I said.

"That's okay, I'll remember," she assured me, "It will be easy to ask them; the convertibles will have the tops down and everybody's windows will be rolled down." This young automobile photographer had it all figured out.

Perhaps the two phrases heard most often in Reno during "Hot August Nights" were, "Cool car!" and "What year?"

The informal parade of highly polished collectibles rolled past. Somehow it seemed oddly organized, by instinct, each car's driver keeping a modest pace and distance from the others. There was no tailgating, no impulsive lane changing, and no obscene gestures were exchanged. Clearly, all the car owners and drivers were very proud and protective of their own vehicles, and had a high degree of respect for their fellow "cruisers."

"Here comes a '52 Cadillac convertible," Tori Lou exclaimed. "It looks spooky." The car was dark gray, with a dull finish, not as polished as most of the others. We nicknamed it "The Ghost Car."

"Here's another '57 Chevy," she said, "Look at the cool green and white two-tone paint job!"

"Nice car!" I yelled to the driver.

Back came the usual smile, thumbs up, and "thanks" from the occupants.

"Wow, look at this yellow Ford pickup," Tori Lou exclaimed, "check out those flames painted on the front!"

"Nice truck!" I yelled, "What year?"

"Fifty-five!" the person in the passenger seat hollered back, "thanks!"

So it went for over an hour.

"Nice car!"

"What year?"

"Fifty-two!"

"Nice car!"

"Thanks!"

"Nice car! What year?"

"Sixty-three! Thanks!"

Plymouths, Cadillacs, Fords and Chevys. Cropped and chopped, dropped and stock. Later we learned there were over 5,000 collectible cars in town for "Hot August Nights" including over 1,500 from California.

After exhausting the battery in the digital camera, we decided to hang it up for the night. On the way back to our hotel, I asked Tori Lou, "So, what was your favorite?"

"The '55 Chevy Shorty, I think," she replied, "but I really liked a lot of them!"

The "Shorty" was one of the last cars we saw that night; a shiny, bright red 1955 Chevrolet

Sedan Delivery (formal name for a station wagon without windows).

It had undergone an "extreme makeover," with a couple of feet chopped out of its mid-section, making it shorter than the stock model. It was a real eye-catcher.

Our visit to Reno was a part of the trip that would bring back some of the most vivid visual memories. Tori Lou was in a fantasyland.

Shined up super cars were cruising past, with the neon lights of the "Biggest Little City in the World" providing a brilliant backdrop. It was a car buff's paradise!

Chapter Thirty-Nine

It was Wednesday, August 4th, when we pulled out of Reno and started across Nevada. It's approximately four-hundred miles from Reno to the Utah state line. We weren't sure how far we'd get. Looking at the map, Tori Lou read of names off towns where we might stop for the night.

"Winnemucca, Battle Mountain; no, that's only half way," she said, as we got up to freeway speed on Interstate 80 and passed through Reno's neighboring city, Sparks. "Elko, maybe; I don't know," she said.

Boring, but beautiful, might be a way to describe the scenery across the widest part of Nevada traversed by I-80. Driving across the wide open desert plains with the majestic mountains off in the distance, gave us a chance to relax, set the cruise control and enjoy the sunshine. Quite a contrast from the neon-lit car show we'd experienced the night before.

"Only three days and we'll be home," I said to Tori Lou.

"Yep," she replied. I could tell she was still tired from being up late taking pictures of cars on Virginia Street in Reno.

"Are you kind of anxious to see your mom and friends?" I asked.

"Uhhuh," she replied. It seemed she was not awake enough for any thought-provoking discussion. That is, until . . . the cell phone rang.

Out in the middle of nowhere, I answered my cell phone, and heard a small voice say, "Is Tori there?"

"It's for you," I said, handing the phone to Tori Lou.

"Hey, whazzup?" she said smiling. It was Chris, her thirteen-year-old friend, from down the street in Loma Linda.

Suddenly, her conversational skills increased dramatically. "Yeah, I'm in the middle of the desert in Nevada. We saw sooo many cool cars last night in Reno. You wouldn't believe it. I took a lot of pictures. Have you seen Sebastian? Really? You've been taking him for walks? Awesome! Yeah. Really? Yeah. Uhhuh. Yeah. Okay, bahhh!" Tori Lou said, handing me the cell phone, having concluded the rapid-fire dialogue.

"So, how's Chris doing?" I asked.

"Good," she answered.

"I heard you say Chris has been walking Sebastian?" I prompted.

"Yup," she said.

"Check out those big mountains way over there," I said, as she turned on the CD player.

She selected CD 1, Track 8: "Come Fly With Me" by Michael Buble.

By now, we had both learned all the words to that and several other songs on the CD. We loved to sing along, with the sun shining, and the cruise control holding steady at 83 miles an hour.

At a rest stop somewhere around Elko, near Humboldt National Forest, we asked someone, whose car bore a Nevada license plate, where would be a good place to stop for the night.

She told us, "Wendover. It's about ninety miles or so, right at the Utah border. They have a couple of nice hotels and casinos there."

About two hours later, we reached Wendover.

The woman, who'd told us that it was right at the border, wasn't kidding! We saw a sign that said, "Welcome to Utah." Then, seconds after crossing the state line, we turned onto the exit ramp and did a cloverleaf turn right back into Nevada!

We pulled into the Wendover Nugget Hotel and Casino. Entering the large, rather well-appointed lobby, we approached the reception desk. We were the only people in the lobby except for the clerk.

"Can we get a no-smoking room, with two beds?" I asked.

"Sure," the clerk said. "It'll be twenty-nine, ninety-nine."

"I beg your pardon," I said. I was used to paying three to five times that for a hotel room.

"Unless you want a room with double doors that open out onto the swimming pool area," she added. "That's ten dollars more; thirty-nine, ninety-nine."

"We'll take it," I said, wondering why the price was so low.

"We're like . . . a weekend place," the young clerk explained. "We get pretty busy on the weekends, full sometimes, but today's Wednesday. We had dinner in the Nugget Restaurant and we were two of only a handful of customers."

Later we went swimming and we were the only ones in the pool. Wendover is not far from Salt Lake City and I figured out that the Nugget must draw a lot of weekend gamblers from that area. The hotel pool was rather small, and it was a bit chilly that night. We'd gotten a little spoiled by the Southern California weather. But, it was nice to have a swimming pool all to ourselves.

Tori Lou probably would have preferred to have a few of her buddies in the pool to splash around with. All of a sudden, we were no longer alone.

"Yikes, it's a bat!" I yelled as a fluttery little winged warrior zigzagged and zoomed down near our heads.

Tori Lou's head disappeared! She had submerged faster than a bobber on a fishing line hit by a twelve pound walleye. About fifteen seconds later she surfaced. "Is it gone?" she asked, looking around.

"I think so," I said tentatively, "no, look out, here he comes!"

Plop! Tori Lou's head disappeared again, even more quickly.

As she re-surfaced, she said, "Did the bat really come back? Or, did you just make that up?"

"Look out!" I shouted.

Plop! Down again.

That went on for several more "bat attacks," all of which were phony. The bat had long since left the area. When we both began to shiver from the cold water, and from laughing, we decided to turn in for the night.

"It was nice to visit Utah today . . . for about, what was it, twenty seconds?" I said, as we headed toward the ten dollar doors that opened to our hotel room.

Chapter Forty

Thursday morning, August 5th, we were back on Interstate 80, and immediately entered Utah, for the second time in two days. The highway traversed up a sizeable hill and, as we reached the summit, an unexpected sight was revealed to us. A seemingly endless expanse of white was illuminated by the morning sun. We had reached the Great Salt Lake Desert. Interstate 80 strung itself out ahead of us, in a perfectly straight line, as far as the eye could see.

"Somewhere around here are the Bonneville Salt Flats," I told Tori Lou. "It's where all the land speed records have been set."

"Really?" she said, looking around as if she would see Craig Breedlove, former record holder, driving by at 600 miles per hour in his super-powered car, the "Spirit of America."

We did see a sign that said, "Bonneville Salt Flats, Next Exit," but we didn't see any racing cars. The salt flats invite speed, and I put the Mitsubishi to the test. I had the cruise control set higher than the temperature reading that day.

We crossed the salt flats, in record time; at least record time for a guy from Wisconsin who, back home, seldom exceeded the speed limit.

Just West of Salt Lake City, there appeared on the horizon a large conglomerate of buildings that looked like a factory.

As we got closer, I could see that it was a Morton Salt Company plant. We were nearing Grantsville, Utah, one of several places in the world where Morton harvests salt to put in those familiar blue packages bearing a picture of a little girl with an umbrella and the slogan, "When it Rains, it Pours."

"Look, Tori Lou, there's the Morton Salt factory," I said.

"Zzzz," she replied. She was fast asleep. The monotony of the salty desert drive had knocked her out.

Just outside Salt Lake City, she woke up in time to see the Great Salt Lake up close. For several miles, Interstate 80 runs right alongside the lake. As we got closer to the city, the terrain changed noticeably. Now, we could see mountains and trees. It was nice to see something besides salt!

Interstate 80 winds through the city and, from the freeway, we could see the Mormon Tabernacle off in the distance, as well as some of the venues where the 2002 Winter Olympics were held. Not far outside the city, we could see some of the slopes where skiing events took place. Sixty miles or so further, Utah was in the rearview mirror.

We were in the least populated of all the fifty states; the only state to feature a man on a bucking bronco on its license plates; the first state to give women the right to vote; and the home of Yellowstone, the world's first National Park.

We were in Wyoming; and we were determined to "make it to Cheyenne by nightfall." Sounds like a line from a western movie.

The Great Divide Basin is an expansive desert area, punctuated by high buttes and rolling sand dunes, sagebrush and patches of purple larkspur. By early afternoon, we had crossed the Great Divide.

The Rocky Mountains of Wyoming are beautiful, and for Tori Lou, these were the biggest mountains she'd seen since we left Southern California. For me, the Colorado Rockies, which I traversed on my trip three months earlier, were more dramatic.

The highway seemed to have sharper turns and there were more tunnels on the route further to the South. But then, maybe I was just getting used to driving in mountains.

It was a long drive across Wyoming and I started getting serious about stopping for the night around Laramie.

"It's not that much further, Dad," Tori Lou said, "We can make it to Cheyenne."

We pulled in at sunset, just like in the movies; and tied the trusty convertible up to a hitching post right in front of the *Wingate Inn*.

We went to dinner at a nearby *Outback Steakhouse* and ordered a couple of appetizers, instead of entrees. Mozzarella sticks and onion rings had always been among Tori Lou's favorites, but she hardly ate a bite.

"Are you okay?" I asked, "You haven't eaten anything."

"I'm fine," she replied, "Just tired, I think. We did almost four-hundred miles today."

I didn't say anything, but I was thinking that she might be excited about being home in less than forty-eight hours.

Suddenly, she sat up straight in the booth and said, "I forgot to get a T-shirt for Joe!"

A couple of weeks earlier, in Loma Linda, we had gone shopping for souvenir T-shirts for Tori Lou's friends back home in Wisconsin. We found the best selection, and price, at a Walgreen's store.

Tori Lou picked out "California" T-shirts for her mom, her older sister, Jen, and her buddies, Jessica, Taz, Sturgis and Tony. But, somehow she had forgotten her friend, Joe.

As we were on our way back to the hotel, to turn in for the night, she came up with the solution.

"I'll just get him a 'Nebraska' T-shirt. He won't care. We'll pick one up at a truck stop tomorrow. He'll love it."

Chapter Forty-One

We got up at 7 A.M. Friday, August 6th. Our goal was to make it to Omaha, or at least to Lincoln, Nebraska, by the end of the day. From either of these cities, we could make it all the way home to Madison in one day. We departed Cheyenne without having breakfast.

About an hour into Nebraska, I thought Tori Lou might be getting hungry. "Want to stop for some breakfast?" I asked.

"Yeah, I really want a waffle!" she responded brightly. Apparently, whatever had caused her to lose her appetite the night before was no longer a factor.

As luck would have it, at the next interchange there was a Perkins Restaurant. We were familiar with Perkins, having been to the one in Madison. "They have good waffles; let's go there," Tori Lou said, as I turned onto the exit ramp.

But, when we walked in to the restaurant, we saw there were perhaps a dozen parties ahead of us waiting to get a table.

"This could take a long time, Lou," I said, "maybe we should go somewhere else, on down the line. Otherwise, we might not even make it to Lincoln tonight."

"Okay, sure," she said, obviously disappointed. She had really been looking forward to a waffle.

After leaving Perkins with an empty stomach, Tori Lou wasn't saying a word as we headed East on Interstate 80, and she was kind of hunched down in her seat. Her body language was saying loud and clear, "You should have waited for that waffle, Dad."

The road ahead looked barren and lifeless. I was convinced that we would not be seeing any sign of civilization, let alone a waffle, for hours.

I thought, "Please, let there be a waffle place along this highway!"

"You doing okay, Lou?" I said, breaking the silence.

"Yeah, I'm fine," she said.

Her body language continued to say, "I'm hungry."

"I know you were really looking forward to breakfast; we'll stop at the next place we see," I assured her.

The road ahead looked desolate. I kept thinking, "There has to be something up ahead."

Suddenly, there it was! I thought, at first, "It must be a mirage."

The sign said, "Grandma Max's Restaurant;" the menu said, "Homemade Belgian Waffles, our specialty!"

Hallelujah! Thank you, Grandma Max!

We finished breakfast and got back on the Interstate. Tori Lou sat up straight, and sang along with Michael Buble. Whatever Grandma Max put into her waffles seemed to do the trick.

To shield our eyes from the sun, we were both wearing baseball caps. Mine was a green cap that said "Loma Linda University" and Tori Lou was wearing her favorite, the white cap with a red, Hurley logo on the front.

It was the hat she'd chosen at the skateboard shop in Redlands, on her second day in California. She had worn it almost every day since.

We were almost halfway across Nebraska when I saw a sign that referred to Lexington.

"Look, Tori Lou," I said, pointing to the sign, "That's the town where I stayed my first night out, on my way to California."

"Oh, yeah," she said, "where you were, when I called you on the cell phone." She rose up slightly to get a better look.

Then, it happened. Whoosh! Her favorite white baseball cap was suddenly a little white dot in the rearview mirror.

"I'm afraid it's a goner, Lou," I said sadly. "There's no way we can stop, or turn around, out here on the Interstate."

"It's okay," she said, "I've got a lot of other hats." She was being a trooper, but I knew she felt bad.

"Maybe we could go online when we get home," I suggested, "And order the same hat."

"Yeah, maybe," she said, "Oh, we have to remember to get a T-shirt for Joe! Watch for truck stops."

Apparently there would be no extended grieving period in remembrance of the baseball cap. I think she was just trying to forget about it.

It was just a hat, I thought to myself. But, it was also an example of how something you care about can be lost, in a flash, and without warning. Something unexpected can come along; and something you love is suddenly gone.

Just like that. It can be a gust of wind, a misspoken word, an accident . . . an illness.

As I focused on watching for truck stops, I reflected, once again, on how lucky I was to have found Loma Linda and to have been able to spend several weeks with Tori Lou. Behind my cool shades, I blinked away a tear, as I realized our journey was nearly over.

The next day, we would be back in Wisconsin. It would no longer be "just the two of us." Tori Lou would return to spend the majority of time at her mom's house; school would be starting soon; friends would become her main focus.

"Dad! There's a SAPP Brothers!" Tori Lou announced.

I pulled into the huge truck stop, one of several operated by SAPP Brothers across Nebraska. We needed gas, so I filled the tank. Then we went inside to look for a T-shirt for Joe. We found the perfect one almost immediately.

"This is it, Dad!" Tori Lou said, "Perfect for Joe!" She held up the shirt. Across the front, in block letters, it read, "Nebraska" and below was a single ear of bright yellow corn. Joe has a keen sense of humor, and we felt he would enjoy having a shirt from the Cornhusker State, when everyone else got a shirt from California.

"The kids who get the California shirts will be jealous," I cautioned Tori Lou.

"Yeah, right," said Tori Lou, grinning as she held the shirt up again to get another look. Folding the shirt and handing it to me, she turned to another rack.

"Look! They have *Sturgis* shirts," Tori Lou said, holding up a baby blue, yet kind of macho-looking T-shirt, emblazoned with the word *Sturgis* and a picture of some leather-clad, rugged-looking bikers, confidently perched on their Harleys.

It was less than a week before the start of the "65ᵗʰ Annual Black Hills Motorcycle Rally" in Sturgis, South Dakota, not far from where we were.

"Sturgis will love this! Can I get it for him?" she pleaded.

Sturgis, a friend and classmate of hers, was named after the town in South Dakota because his dad and mom were avid bikers who regularly attend the famous summertime rally.

We took both shirts to the check out counter.

"Can we get some sunflower seeds?" Tori Lou asked.

"Sure, as long as you don't let the seeds fly into the back seat when you spit them out," I said.

"I'll be careful!"

We pulled into Lincoln, Nebraska just after dark. Too tired to make it to Omaha, we found a room at a Holiday Inn Express and decided to eat dinner in our room. There was a KFC about fifty yards from the hotel, so I walked over to get some chicken, mashed potatoes and gravy.

"Hey, if we can eat at an Italian restaurant in Chinatown, and eat Chinese food in Little Italy," I said to Tori Lou, "we can eat Kentucky Fried Chicken in Nebraska."

We watched TV for awhile, and then dozed off to the sound of 18-wheelers growling along the nearby Interstate.

Chapter Forty-Two

It was the last day of our journey, Saturday, August 7th, 2004. In four days we had been to four state capitals; Sacramento, Salt Lake City, Cheyenne and Lincoln.

And, on this final day, we'd see two more; Des Moines and Madison. Six state capitals in five days, and without getting on a plane.

We left Lincoln, made it through Omaha, and crossed the Missouri river into Iowa. The corn was tall and richly green. While we were basking in the California sun, there had been plenty of rain in the Midwest and it had been good for the crops.

Interstate 80 draws a straight line across the map of Iowa–the land of one small town after another. We passed little places like Walnut, Adair, and Dexter; Casey, Booneville, Malcom; and one big place, Des Moines.

We left Interstate 80, just before Iowa City, and got onto Route 151 and headed north through the Amana Colonies to Cedar Rapids, where we passed St. Luke's Hospital. I said, "Tori Lou, I think that's the hospital where your mom was born."

Tori Lou grabbed the cell phone and immediately called Madison.

"Hey, Mom," she said, "you won't believe this! We just drove by the hospital where we think you were born! St. Luke's? Yeah. I just saw it."

On a cue from me, Tori Lou added, "And, it's still there!"

From the driver's seat, I could hear her mom laughing on the cell phone.

"We'll make it to Madison tonight," Tori Lou told her mom, "but, it might be late. I'll sleep at Dad's tonight and he can bring me home in the morning, if that's okay. We have to unpack the car and sort out our stuff and that will take awhile."

Although she was anxious to see her daughter, Laura agreed with the plan. I was glad, because I hoped that Tori Lou could be with me the first night back home. I missed her already, and she was still in the car beside me.

It was a strange feeling, pulling into the driveway of my condo, and pushing the garage door opener, which hadn't been out of the glove compartment in three months. It worked!

The door went up, revealing our bikes, with partially deflated tires, a snow shovel hanging on the wall; and all of the things that we'd put in the garage, because there was no place else to put them.

There were plastic flower pots, an old rolled up area rug, my cat's "traveling cage," and boxes of miscellaneous items which I'd never unpacked, after moving into the condo, over six years before. The place was the same. But somehow things always seem somewhat strange, when you first come home after a fairly long time away.

In the foyer stood the two large cardboard boxes of things we had shipped home, via FedEx, from California.

"I told you they'd get here before us," I said to Tori Lou.

"Yeah, my shoes are in there!" she said as she ran up the stairs, went directly to her room, and plopped down on the bottom bunk of her bed. "This feels good," she said.

"It is good to be home," I agreed, letting out a deep breath.

I flashed back, in my mind, to those many times I'd plopped down on that very same bed, having returned from a trip with my mom and stepfather. My mother, Minnie, had purchased the bunk beds for me when I was about six years old. The beds had been in storage for years, until Tori Lou insisted on having them for her room.

While she lay on the bottom bunk, Tori Lou could read the hieroglyphics scrawled in pencil and crayon on the wooden slats which supported the top bed.

One is Ancient: "Billy Vancil" - in shaky, little-kid cursive. One is Modern: "Tori Lou Vancil" - in assertive, pre-teen handwriting. Both are priceless.

I couldn't resist telling Tori Lou how I remembered when my buddy, Steve (now my stock broker, living in Mississippi), slept over at my house.

One time, Steve and I took a discarded roll of cardboard (the kind used for wrapping paper) and fashioned a pulley made out of Tinker

Toys and string. Using this device, we would pass notes up and down between the lower and upper bunks.

In more modern times, Tori Lou and her friends use "text messaging" on their cell phones.

Nonetheless, the story fascinated Lou. "Do we have any cardboard rolls?" she asked, "That sounds cool; I want to try it sometime."

I didn't ask her if she'd like to do her homework on the back of a wooden shovel, writing with a piece of coal, as Abe and I used to do.

Chapter Forty-Three

Tori Lou fell asleep that night with the TV on, as she always does. As I came into her room to turn off the late night cartoon show, I paused to look around.

I smiled as I gazed at the posters on the wall, her bubble gum-machine bank, and messy desk. There was a pile of stuffed animals she'd collected over the years. And right at the top of the heap, there he sat! My first teddy bear. The one I got for Christmas, when I was two years old, and had given to Tori Lou some time back.

She'd had a hard time believing, when I'd told her that I actually remember coming down the stairway, over 60 years ago, at my grandparents' farmhouse near Kewanee, Illinois, and seeing "Teddy" under the tree.

He had a small, red tongue which I chewed off the very first day. Later when his eyes fell off, my mother replaced them with sewn-on buttons.

That bear has been all over the USA. When my folks and I took a trip, Teddy came along. I'm not sure why he didn't make the trip to

Loma Linda. I just forgot to take him. I didn't try to explain; he had always been very forgiving. Imagine, having your eyes sewn on!

As I lay in bed that night, I was filled with mixed emotions. I felt happiness, because I had completed the proton treatment and felt good physically, but I also felt sadness, because the summertime odyssey of Bill and Tori Lou was ending.

The doctors, both in California and Wisconsin, would keep watch on my condition, by performing checkups and PSA tests regularly, and there was no reason to think that the treatments had not been successful.

I assumed a positive attitude, since the time I was diagnosed with prostate cancer back in early February. And I was determined to maintain that positive attitude after returning home. But, I could feel a letdown coming on. I was at "home," but feeling "homesick" at the same time.

I fell asleep thinking of Tori Lou and I returning to Southern California from time-to-time, so we can see our friends, and she can surf again at Newport Beach and skate again at Chino.

It took a long time to fall asleep, as I also thought of taking other trips with Tori Lou, to different places in the world. I tried to tell myself, "This is not the end of our travels; it's the beginning."

Then, I faced the realization that perhaps, as she grew older, Tori Lou would not *want* to travel with Dad. We had talked about it some, and her quick answer was, as I expected, "If I can bring a friend."

Covering my tracks, I had asked her, "Well, what if you invited a friend, who wasn't able to go, would you still go, with just me?"

"Sure," she said, giving me a puzzled look, which I loosely interpreted as, "You're my Dad. Why wouldn't I want to go?"

I had learned that a puzzled look from Tori Lou is bankable.

Chapter Forty-Four

The journey had started on Sunday, May 9th and was ending on Sunday, August 8th. It was exactly three months since Tori Lou and I said goodbye in the driveway in front of her mom's condo.

As soon as we finished unpacking, which we'd started the night before, and had sorted out our things, we would be returning to that driveway.

"Make three piles," I said, "one pile of things you will take with you to your mom's, one pile of things you'll leave here, and one pile of things you'll leave here for me to wash."

She laughed, and added, "And, one pile for the souvenirs I brought back."

We pulled up in front of Laura's condo about 9:30 A.M. There were the expected hugs and tears, and then Tori Lou broke into some serious souvenir distribution.

Some of the presentations would have to wait until her friends arrived later in the day for the "Welcome Home, Tori Lou" get-together. An event planned, for the most part, by her.

After spending an hour or so listening to Tori Lou tell her sister and her mom all about the trip, I prepared to leave. And somehow I managed to keep a smiling face, as I said, "Give me a hug, Lou. I'll see you soon."

It was the same kind of long hug, which seemed short, that we had shared three months earlier. I drove home forcing myself to think ahead, not back.

"I'll have to hook up my computer first thing tomorrow and get back into the work routine," I told myself. "This is good. I need to get back into the routine. I really do."

The next day, while putting my office back together, I contacted some of my friends and clients to let them know I was back in Madison.

Some people, with whom I'd been working on projects by long distance, didn't even know I had been gone. I explained it to those I felt had the time to listen.

Over the next two weeks, I didn't see Tori Lou, but I talked to her on the phone and exchanged some emails.

She was very busy getting back in the swing of things with her friends; showing them her improved skateboarding skills, telling them about her trip, and trying to make the most of what was left of summer.

School would be starting on September 1st.

Chapter Forty-Five

On Friday night, August 20th. I picked up Tori Lou at about 11:00 P.M. at the bowling alley, where she had gone with her friends for the weekly ritual known as *"Cyber Bowling."*

Each Friday, from 9 P.M. until Midnight, the bowling lanes are illuminated by strobe lights, laser beams and mirror balls. The lanes remain mostly empty, while kids talk, eat, and occasionally, bowl.

The next morning, Saturday, August 21st, Tori Lou and I went shopping for "Back to School" supplies and clothes. Our first top was at Office Depot, to get paper, pencils, glue, notebooks, calculator, markers, and every thing else on the list, which had been provided by her teacher.

The shopping for supplies was accented by periodic yawns and some slumping by my late-night bowler.

Approximately $85 later, we had everything on the list, and we were heading for the mall. We had planned to get Tori Lou some new jeans for school, maybe a top or two, and a bunch of new socks. We purchased socks at Penney's, but for the jeans, we needed to go to a different store.

"It's right down this way, Dad," Tori Lou said, for some reason, not nearly as tired as she had been while in Office Depot.

"There it is! Pac Sun!" she pointed to the store front, which was decked out in California paraphernalia, featuring surf boards and palm trees.

"I thought you usually get jeans for school at Penney's," I said, as we walked into the store filled with surfing and skateboarding brands.

"Penney's is okay," she explained, "but, these fit me better. They have the same brand that I bought at the mall in California!"

After picking out a couple of pairs of jeans and a top, Tori Lou informed me that she really needed a new pair of skateboard shoes.

"Didn't you just get a pair, when we were in Loma Linda?" I reminded her.

"Yeah, but look," she was wearing the California shoes and held one up to show me the hole she'd worn in it already.

"All right," I said, "see if they have your size."

Chapter Forty-Six

As Tori Lou was trying on what would be her fourth or fifth pair of skateboard shoes of the summer, something made me glance up toward the ceiling of the store. High on a shelf, just above where Tori Lou was sitting, I spotted it.

"Look up there, Lou," I said, pointing to the shelf near the ceiling.

"My hat!" she exclaimed.

It was a white baseball cap with a red "Hurley" logo on the front, a replica of the one that was abruptly confiscated by a barbaric gust of wind, somewhere on the Great Plains of Nebraska.

"Do you want to get it?" I asked.

"Well, those hats are kind of expensive, and I've already got all this other stuff," she replied.

"But, it's a pretty important hat, don't you think?" I asked her. "It's just like the one you wore for most of our trip."

After a moment of contemplation, she admitted, "Yeah, I want to get it."

"I thought so," I nodded.

The clerk had to use a long pole to reach the hat, because it was perched up so high on the store shelf.

Arm-in-arm, Tori Lou and I left the mall with Pac Sun jeans, socks from Penney's, a reincarnated Hurley hat, yet *another* pair of skateboard shoes . . . and each other.

I mused that Tori Lou's journey into 8th grade, and beyond, was about to begin.

Just how far might her many talents take her?

Thanks to the journey to Loma Linda, her Dad will be around to find out.

God willing.

Post Script

On November 29th, 2004, Tori Lou's fourteenth birthday, not long before this book went to print, Bill and Tori Lou both received some good news.

Having completed his four-month post-treatment checkup, Bill learned that his PSA score was *less than* 0.05, down from 7.15 when first diagnosed.

Tori Lou, having completed the first semester of eighth grade, learned that she had made the honor roll, with an A-minus average.

Regarding both scores, Bill commented, "It pays to do your homework."

He added, "By making an effort to learn all I could about the various methods of treatment for prostate cancer, I was able to choose the type with which I was most comfortable."

Every man faced with this challenge should do the same. Whatever his choice of treatment, it will stand a better chance of success if he fully believes in it.

Continue the Journey

www.dontfearthebigdogs.com

The official book website. See photos taken on the Journey to Loma Linda; get information relevant to the book and its author; and find links to related websites.

www.protonbob.com

Website of the international prostate cancer support group, "Brotherhood of the Balloon." Learn more about proton therapy and read testimonials from many patients

www.llu.edu/proton

Web page for the Loma Linda University Medical Center Proton Treatment Center. A great place to start learning more about proton radiation treatment.

At time of this book's publication, proton therapy was available in the USA only at Loma Linda University in California; Massachusetts General Hospital in Boston; and at Indiana University in Bloomington. Facilities were scheduled to open in early 2006 at M. D. Anderson Cancer Treatment Center in Houston and at University of Florida Shands in Jacksonville.

To arrange media interviews, personal appearances, or any special assistance the author may be able to provide, send email to Bill Vancil at <u>bill@dontfearthebigdogs.com</u>

To order more copies of this book contact

TATE PUBLISHING, LLC

127 East Trade Center Terrace
Mustang, Oklahoma 73064

(888) 361 - 9473

Tate Publishing, LLC

www.tatepublishing.com